AF393124

CONTENTS

IMMUNE BOOSTING SMOOTHIES

Coco-maca Smoothie

Servings: 1
Cooking Time: 5 Minutes
Ingredients:
- 1 cup coconut milk,
- 1 banana (fresh or frozen)
- A handful of mixed berries
- 1 teaspoon coconut oil
- ½ teaspoon vanilla extract
- ½ tablespoon Cacao powder
- 1 tablespoon Chia seeds
- ½ teaspoon raw, organic honey or liquid stevia (optional)

Directions:
1. Load your blender with all the ingredients and pulse it up until there are no more lumps.

Nutrition Info: (Per Serving): Calories-285, Fat-7 g, Protein-21 g, Carbohydrates-40 g

Banana-avocado Smoothie

Servings: 1
Cooking Time: 2 Minutes
Ingredients:
- 2 kiwis, peeled and chopped
- 1 large banana, chopped
- 2 cups spinach
- 2 tablespoons avocado flesh
- A pinch of cinnamon powder
- ½ cup filtered water

Directions:
1. Fill up your blender jar with the fruits, greens, and water and blend until well combined.
2. Sprinkle a dash of cinnamon powder on top and serve.

Nutrition Info: (Per Serving): Calories-300, Fat-8.3 g, Protein- 6.3 g, Carbohydrates -60.6 g

Berry Mint Smoothie

Servings: 1
Cooking Time: 5 Minutes
Ingredients:
- 1 cup strawberries, fresh or frozen
- 1 cup unsweetened almond milk
- 2 kale leaves, chopped
- 1 tablespoon Chia seeds
- 1 tablespoon lemon zest
- 1 teaspoon raw, organic honey
- 1-2 sprigs of fresh mint
- 1-2 ice cubes (optional)

Directions:
1. To you blender, add all the above ingredient and pulse until smooth.

Citrus Spinach Immune Booster

Servings: 2
Cooking Time: 5 Minutes
Ingredients:
- 1 orange, peeled, deseeded and chopped
- 1 lime, peeled, deseeded and chopped
- A small handful of spinach leaves, washed
- 1-2 peaches, peeled and chopped
- 2 carrots, peeled and chopped
- 1 ½ cups almond milk (unsweetened)

Directions:
1. Dump all the ingredients into the blender and whip it up until the smoothie is thick and creamy.
Nutrition Info: (Per Serving): Calories-145, Fat-2g, Protein- 4 g, Carbohydrates- 30 g

Cacao- Spirulina And Berry Booster

Servings: 1
Cooking Time: 5 Minutes
Ingredients:
- 1 banana, (fresh or frozen)
- 1 cup coconut milk
- 1 cup strawberries (fresh or frozen)
- 1 cup mixed greens
- ½ cup blueberries (frozen)
- 1 teaspoon cacao powder
- 1 teaspoon Spirulina powder
- ½ tablespoon coconut oil
- A large pinch of cinnamon powder
- 1 teaspoon of raw, organic honey,
- 1 tablespoon of any super food of your choice 9 mace, goji berry, bee pollen, aloe, hemp etc.)

Directions:
1. Load your smoothie blender with all the mentioned ingredients and pulse it on high speed for 2 minutes.
2. Pour into a glass and enjoy.
Nutrition Info: (Per Serving): Calories- 390, Fat- 18 g , Protein- 15 g, Carbohydrates- 50 g

Orange Coco Smoothie

Servings: 2
Cooking Time: 10 Minutes
Ingredients:

- 1 cup freshly squeezed orange juice
- 6 California tangerines, peeled and chopped
- 1 cup mixed greens
- 2 teaspoons freshly grated ginger root
- Juice of 2 freshly squeezed lemons
- 1 ½ cups of coconut milk/ coconut water (your choice)
- 4 teaspoons pure coconut oil
- 2 tablespoons Chia seeds
- 4 teaspoons raw organic honey
- 1 tablespoons any super food of your choice

Directions:

1. To your blender jar, add all the ingredients in the given order and whirr it up for 90 seconds or until done.

Nutrition Info: (Per Serving): Calories-267, Fat-1.3 g, Protein-5.3 g, Carbohydrates- 68.4 g

Blueberry Peach Smoothie

Servings: 1
Cooking Time: 5 Minutes
Ingredients:

- 1 cup almond milk
- 1 cup peach, cubed (fresh or frozen)
- A handful of blueberries (fresh or frozen)
- 1 cup greens of your choice (kale, spinach)
- 1 tablespoon of Chia seeds
- ½ teaspoon of freshly grated ginger
- 1 tablespoon of any super food of your choice
- 1 tablespoon coconut oil

Directions:

1. Add all the ingredients to the blender jar except the coconut oil and process for 1 minute.
2. Then pour in the oil and blend again for 30 seconds and serve.

Nutrition Info: (Per Serving): Calories- 280, Fat- 18 g, Protein- 3 g, Carbohydrates- 34 g

Berrilicious Chiller

Servings: 2
Cooking Time: 5 Minutes
Ingredients:

- 1 ½ cup mixed berries (fresh or frozen)
- 1 tablespoon freshly squeezed lemon juice
- 6 ounces of unsweetened almond milk
- 2 teaspoons of freshly grated ginger
- 1 tablespoon flax seeds
- 1 ½ tablespoons of raw organic honey
- A handful of ice cubes

Directions:

1. Add all the ingredients into your blender and process until smooth and frothy.

2. Serve and enjoy immediately.
Nutrition Info: (Per Serving): Calories- 110, Fat-1.5 g, Protein- 1 g, Carbs-26 g

Apple-kiwi Slush

Servings: 1
Cooking Time: 2 Minutes
Ingredients:
- 2 kiwis, peeled and chopped
- 1 apple, cored and chopped
- Cups baby spinach
- 1 large carrot, peeled and chopped
- 4 oz. filtered water

Directions:
1. Load your blender with all the ingredients and process it on high until thick and frothy.
Nutrition Info: (Per Serving): Calories-200, Fat-1.2 g, Protein- 4.8 g, Carbohydrates-51 g

Popoye's Pear Smoothie For Kids

Servings: 1
Cooking Time: 5 Minutes
Ingredients:
- 1 pear, diced
- ½ avocado
- 1 kiwi, peeled and chopped
- A handful of baby spinach
- A few mixed berries

Directions:
1. Wash all the produce thoroughly and add them to the blender.
2. Process it for 1 minute or until well combined.
3. Serve.
Nutrition Info: (Per Serving): Calories-320, Fat-15 g, Protein-4 g, Carbohydrates-50 g

Creamy Pink Smoothie

Servings: 2
Cooking Time: 5 Minutes
Ingredients:
- 2 cups strawberries (fresh or frozen)
- 2 tablespoon cashew butter
- 1 ½ cup of almond milk (unsweetened)
- 2 tablespoons rolled oats
- 1 teaspoon vanilla extract
- 1 teaspoon raw organic honey
- A pinch of cinnamon power
- 1 teaspoon of cashew flakes (garnish)

Directions:
1.   Place all the ingredients in your blender and run it on high for 1 minute.
2.   Pour into serving glasses and top it with a sprinkle of cashew flakes.
3.   Enjoy!

Double Decker Smoothie

Servings: 2
Cooking Time: 10 Minutes
Ingredients:
- For 1st layer (orange):
- 1 persimmon, quartered
- The juice of 1 lime
- 1 cup coconut milk
- 1 mango, peeled and chopped
- 1 tablespoon almond butter
- A pinch of cayenne pepper
- ½ teaspoon turmeric powder
- For 2nd layer (pink)
- 1 small beetroot, peeled and chopped
- 1 cup mixed berries (fresh or frozen)
- ½ cup filtered water
- 1 small grapefruit, peeled and quartered
- 5-6 fresh mint leaves
- Garnish- mint leaves, 1 teaspoon of Chia seeds

Directions:
1.   Add the ingredients of the first layer into the blender and process it for 1 minute until smooth.
2.   Pour the mixture equally into 2 serving glasses and keep it aside.
3.   In the same blender, add the ingredients of the second layer and process whir it up until and smooth.
4.   Divide this pink mixture equally into the 2 serving glass, above the first layer.
5.   Sprinkle some Chia seeds on top and add a garnish with a mint leaf.
6.   Serve immediately.

Nutrition Info: (Per Serving): Calories-320, Fat-5.2 g, Protein-4.5 g, Carbohydrates-72.7 g

Ultimate Cold And Flu Fighting Smoothie

Servings: 1
Cooking Time: 5 Minutes
Ingredients:
- 1 large banana, fresh or frozen
- 2 oranges, peeled and chopped
- 2 cups baby spinach
- Freshly squeezed juice of ½ lemon
- 2 tablespoon Chia seeds (soaked)
- 1 teaspoon of freshly grated ginger

- ¼ cup of filtered water

Directions:

1. Whizz all the ingredients in the blender until smooth and serve.

Nutrition Info: (Per Serving): Calories- 330, Fat- 5.8 g, Protein-8 g, Carbohydrates-72 g

Strawberry-ginger Tea Smoothie

Servings: 1

Cooking Time: 5 Minutes

Ingredients:

- 1 cup freshly brewed ginger tea (warm or hot)
- ½ cup strawberries, tops removed
- 1 oranges, peeled and chopped
- ½ line, peeled and chopped
- Juice of ½ lemon
- ¼ teaspoon of freshly grated ginger
- 1 clove of garlic
- A pinch of cayenne pepper
- ¼ teaspoon of cinnamon powder
- 1 teaspoon coconut oil
- 2 tablespoons raw, organic honey
- A pinch of sea salt
- 4-5 cubes of ice (optional)

Directions:

1. Prepare a cup of ginger tea and keep it aside.
2. Add all the ingredients into your blender except the tea and process it for a minute.
3. Then add the tea and pulse it for another minute or until well blended.

Nutrition Info: (Per Serving): Calories- 210, fat- 5 g, Protein- 1 g, Carbohydrates- 50 g

DETOX AND CLEANSE SMOOTHIES

Mango Pepper Smoothie

Servings: 2
Cooking Time: 5 Minutes
Ingredients:
- 2 cups fresh coconut water
- 2 cups mango, peeled and chopped
- ¼ cup freshly squeezed lime juice
- A pinch of cayenne pepper
- 1-2 cubes of ice

Directions:
1. Place all the ingredients into the blender and pulse on high for 30 seconds or until the smoothie has reached your desired consistency.

Nutrition Info: (Per Serving): Calories-160, Fat- 0 g, Protein- 3 g, Carbohydrates- 40 g

Very-berry Orange

Servings: 1 Large
Cooking Time: 2 Minutes
Ingredients:
- 1 cup blueberries, fresh or frozen
- 1 cup raspberries, fresh or frozen
- 2 large oranges, peeled and chopped
- A few ice cubes

Directions:
1. Add everything to the blender and process on high for 30 seconds.
2. Pour into glass and serve chilled.

Nutrition Info: (Per Serving): Calories- 132, Fat-0 g, Protein- 2 g, Carbohydrates- 34 g

Strawberry-beet Smoothie

Servings: 2 Large
Cooking Time: 5 Minutes
Ingredients:
- 1 cup unsweetened almond milk
- 1 cup red beet, peeled and chopped
- 1 orange, peeled and chopped
- 3 cups baby spinach, washed
- 1 banana, chopped (fresh or frozen)
- 1 cup strawberries (fresh or frozen)

Directions:
1. Place all the ingredients in your blender jar and blend for 1-2 minutes until smooth.

Nutrition Info: (Per Serving): Calories- 333, Fat- 4 g, Proteins- 9 g, Carbohydrates- 71 g

Green Tea- Berry Smoothie

Servings: 2
Cooking Time: 10 Minutes
Ingredients:
- 1 cup green tea (chilled)
- 1/3 cup raspberries (fresh or frozen)
- 1/3 cup blueberries (fresh or frozen)
- 1/3 cup black berries (fresh or frozen)
- ½ small avocado, peeled and chopped
- 1 cup fresh spinach, washed
- 1/3 cup plain yogurt
- 2 teaspoon of freshly squeezed lemon juice

Directions:
1. First, prepare a cup green tea as usual (sugarless) and let it cool down at room temperature.
2. Then chill it in the refrigerator for a few minutes.
3. After the tea has chilled, pour all the ingredients into the blender jar and whizz it for 1 minute or until the smoothie is thick and creamy.

Nutrition Info: (Per Serving): Calories- 365. Fat- 15 g, Protein-10 g, Carbohydrates- 56.6 g

Blueberry Detox Drink

Servings: 2
Cooking Time: 5 Minutes
Ingredients:
- 1 cup ice
- 2 tablespoons spirulina
- ½ frozen banana, sliced
- 2 cups blueberries, frozen
- 2 cups baby spinach
- 2 cups coconut water

Directions:
1. Add all the ingredients except vegetables/fruits first
2. Blend until smooth
3. Add the vegetable/fruits
4. Blend until smooth
5. Add a few ice cubes and serve the smoothie
6. Enjoy!

Nutrition Info: Calories: 685; Fat: 60g; Carbohydrates: 40g; Protein: 32g

Wheatgrass Detox Smoothie

Servings: 2
Cooking Time: 10 Minutes
Ingredients:
- 3 tablespoons Swiss chard
- 1 banana, peeled
- 3 tablespoons almonds

- 1 teaspoon wheatgrass powder
- 2 kiwis, peeled
- 1 cup ice
- 1 cup of water

Directions:
1. Add all the listed ingredients to blender except kiwis
2. Blend until smooth
3. Add kiwis and blend again
4. Serve chilled and enjoy!

Nutrition Info: Calories: 154; Fat: 6g; Carbohydrates: 24g; Protein: 4g

Kale And Beet 2020 Fusion

Servings: 2
Cooking Time: 5 Minutes
Ingredients:
- ¼ teaspoon cinnamon
- ¼ lemon, juiced
- 1 medium cucumber, cubed
- 4 cups kale, chopped
- 2 medium beets, scrubbed, halved

Directions:
1. Add all the ingredients except vegetables/fruits first
2. Blend until smooth
3. Add the vegetable/fruits
4. Blend until smooth
5. Add a few ice cubes and serve the smoothie
6. Enjoy!

Nutrition Info: Calories: 69; Fat: 0g; Carbohydrates: 16g; Protein: 4g

Apple And Green Slush

Servings: 1
Cooking Time: 2 Minutes
Ingredients:
- 1 granny smith apple, cored and chopped
- 1 large, ripe banana, chopped (fresh or frozen)
- ½ cup Italian flat leaf parsley
- 1 cup collard greens (stems removed)
- 1 teaspoon freshly squeezed lemon juice
- A few cubes of ice

Directions:
1. Add all the ingredients to your blender and blend until smooth.

Nutrition Info: (Per Serving): Calories- 105, Fat- 0 g, Protein- 2 g, Carbohydrates-26 g

Tropical Smoothie

Servings: 3
Cooking Time: 5 Minutes
Ingredients:
- ½ cup mango, chopped (fresh or frozen)
- ½ cup freshly squeezed orange juice
- 1 medium banana (fresh or frozen)
- ½ cup pineapple, chopped
- ¼ cup baby spinach
- ¼ cup kale (stems removed)
- 2 tablespoon freshly squeezed lemon juice
- 1 teaspoon pure coconut oil
- ½ teaspoon freshly grated ginger
- ½ cup filtered water
- A few ice cubes (if needed)

Directions:
1. Place all the ingredients into your blender and whirr it up on high for 1 minute or until done.

Nutrition Info: (Per Serving): Calories- 200, Fat- 5 g, Protein- 2 g, Carbohydrates- 40 g

Avocado Detox Smoothie

Servings: 3
Cooking Time: 10 Minutes
Ingredients:
- 4 cups spinach, chopped
- 1 avocado, chopped
- 3 cups apple juice
- 2 apples, unpeeled, cored and chopped

Directions:
1. Add all the listed ingredients to a blender
2. Blend until you have a smooth and creamy texture
3. Serve chilled and enjoy!

Nutrition Info: Calories: 336; Fat: 13.8g; Carbohydrates: 55.8g; Protein: 3g

Apricot-peach Smoothie

Servings: 2 Small
Cooking Time: 2 Minutes
Ingredients:
- 2 pitted peaches (fresh or frozen)
- 2 pitted apricots (fresh or frozen)
- 2 carrots, peeled and chopped
- 1 cup fresh butter lettuce
- ½ teaspoon of vanilla extract
- ¾ cup of filtered water
- 2-3 cubes of ice (optional)

Directions:
1.   Add all the above listed ingredients into your blender and process until smoothie is thick and frothy.
Nutrition Info: (Per Serving): Calories-233, Fat- 1 g, Protein- 7 g, Carbohydrates- 52 g

Coconut Pineapple Detox Smoothie

Servings: 2
Cooking Time: 10 Minutes
Ingredients:
- 3 tablespoons Swiss Chard
- 2 tablespoons coconut flakes
- 1 tablespoon chia seeds
- 8 tablespoons pineapple, peeled and chopped
- ½ avocado pitted
- 1 orange, peeled
- 1 cup of water
- 1 cup ice

Directions:
1.   Add all the listed ingredients to a blender
2.   Blend until smooth
3.   Serve chilled and enjoy!
Nutrition Info: Calories: 212; Fat: 0g; Carbohydrates: 26g; Protein: 3g

Cinna-melon Detox Smoothie

Servings: 2-3
Cooking Time: 5 Minutes
Ingredients:
- 1 cup watermelon, chopped
- 1 cup dandelion greens, washed and chopped
- 1 large banana, fresh or frozen
- Freshly squeezed juice from ½ lime
- Freshly squeezed juice of 1 lemon
- ½ teaspoon raw organic honey (optional)
- ½ teaspoon turmeric powder
- 1 teaspoon freshly grated ginger powder
- ¼ teaspoon of cinnamon powder
- 8 ounces of filtered water
- 1-2 ice cubes

Directions:
1.   Pour all the ingredients into your blender and process until thick and frothy.
Nutrition Info: (Per Serving): Calories- 182, Fat- 1 g, Protein- 4 g, Carbohydrates- 45 g

Chamomile Ginger Detox Smoothie

Servings: 2
Cooking Time: 10 Minutes
Ingredients:
- 3 tablespoons collard greens
- 1 tablespoon chamomile flowers, dried
- 1 pear, chopped
- 1 cantaloupe, sliced and chopped
- ½ inch ginger, peeled
- ½ lemon, juiced
- 1 cup ice
- 1 cup of water

Directions:
1. Add all the listed ingredients to a blender
2. Blend until smooth
3. Serve chilled and enjoy!

Nutrition Info: Calories: 86; Fat: 0g; Carbohydrates: 22g; Protein: 2g

PROTEIN SMOOTHIES

Healthy Chocolate Milkshake

Servings: 2
Cooking Time: 10 Minutes
Ingredients:
- 1 Scoop Whey isolate chocolate protein powder
- 16 ounces unsweetened almond milk, vanilla
- 1 pack stevia
- ½ cup crushed ice

Directions:
1. Add all the listed ingredients to a blender
2. Blend until you have a smooth and creamy texture
3. Serve chilled and enjoy!

Nutrition Info: Calories: 292; Fat: 25g; Carbohydrates: 4g; Protein: 15g

Sweet Protein And Cherry Shake

Servings: 2
Cooking Time: 5 Minutes
Ingredients:
- 1 cup water
- 3 cups spinach
- 2 bananas, sliced
- 2 cups frozen cherries
- 2 tablespoons cacao powder
- 4 tablespoons hemp seeds, shelled

Directions:
1. Add all the ingredients except vegetables/fruits first
2. Blend until smooth
3. Add the vegetable/fruits
4. Blend until smooth
5. Add a few ice cubes and serve the smoothie
6. Enjoy!

Nutrition Info: Calories: 111; Fat: 3g; Carbohydrates: 9g; Protein: 13g

Mixed Berry Melba

Servings: 3
Cooking Time: 5 Minutes
Ingredients:
- 1 cup low fat plain yogurt
- ½ cup mixed berries (fresh or frozen)
- ½ cup whole strawberries (fresh or frozen)
- 1 small banana, chopped
- 3 teaspoons peanut butter or peanut powder
- 2 teaspoons chia seeds

- 1 teaspoon flaxseeds
- ¼ cup filtered water
- 1-2 ice cubes (optional)

Directions:

1. Dump all the ingredients into the blender and whip it up until the smoothie is thick and creamy.

Nutrition Info: (Per Serving): Calories- 340, Fat- 6.3 g, Protein- 25 g, Carbohydrates- 52 g

Coconut Peach Passion

Servings: 3
Cooking Time: 5 Minutes

Ingredients:

- 1 cup unsweetened coconut milk
- 1 ½ cups peach, pitted and chopped
- ¾ cup plain low fat green yogurt
- ½ cup rolled oats
- 1 large ripe banana, chopped
- ¼ teaspoon vanilla extract
- ¼ cup filtered water
- 2-3 ice cubes

Directions:

1. Whizz up all the ingredients in the high speed blender until smooth and serve immediately.

Nutrition Info: (Per Serving): Calories- 265, Fat- 3.2 g, Protein- 12 g, Carbohydrates- 35 g

Iron And Protein Shake

Servings: 2
Cooking Time: 5 Minutes

Ingredients:

- 2 tablespoons favorite sweetened syrup
- 1 cup water
- ¼ cup hemp seeds
- 2 large bananas, frozen
- 4 cups strawberries, sliced

Directions:

1. Add all the ingredients except vegetables/fruits first
2. Blend until smooth
3. Add the vegetable/fruits
4. Blend until smooth
5. Add a few ice cubes and serve the smoothie
6. Enjoy!

Nutrition Info: Calories: 156; Fat: 14g; Carbohydrates: 1g; Protein: 7g

Berry Dreamsicle Smoothie

Servings: 3 - 4

Cooking Time: 5 Minutes
Ingredients:
- 1 cup whole blueberries (fresh or frozen)
- 1/2 ripe banana, chopped
- ½ cup whole strawberries (fresh or frozen)
- 3 large handfuls of chopped lucent kale
- 1 tablespoon freshly squeezed lemon juice
- 2 tablespoons chia seeds
- ½ cup filtered water
- 3-4 ice cubes

Directions:
1. Whizz all the ingredients in the blender until smooth and serve.

Nutrition Info: (Per Serving): Calories- 400, Fat- 10.5 g, Protein- 17 g, Carbohydrates- 70 g

Pineapple Protein Smoothie

Servings: 3-4
Cooking Time: 5 Minutes
Ingredients:
- 1 ½ cups pineapple, chopped
- 1 medium ripe banana, chopped
- 1 cup plain low fat yogurt
- 1 cup plain unsweetened almond milk
- 2-3 ice cubes

Directions:
1. Place everything in the blender jar, secure the lid and pulse until smooth.

Nutrition Info: (Per Serving): Calories- 170, Fat- 4.7 g, Protein- 11 g, Carbohydrates- 25 g

Almond And Choco-brownie Shake

Servings: 2
Cooking Time: 5 Minutes
Ingredients:
- ½ chocolate brownie bar, chopped
- ¼ cup almonds, chopped
- 1 scoop chocolate whey protein
- 1 cup fat-free milk

Directions:
1. Add all the ingredients except vegetables/fruits first
2. Blend until smooth
3. Add the vegetable/fruits
4. Blend until smooth
5. Add a few ice cubes and serve the smoothie
6. Enjoy!

Nutrition Info: Calories: 578; Fat: 35g; Carbohydrates: 69g; Protein: 17g

Glorious Cinnamon Roll Smoothie

Servings: 1

Cooking Time: 10 Minutes
Ingredients:
- 1 cup unsweetened almond milk
- ½ teaspoon cinnamon
- ¼ teaspoon vanilla extract
- 1 tablespoon chia seeds
- 2 tablespoons vanilla protein powder
- 1 cup ice cubs

Directions:
1. Add all the listed ingredients into your blender
2. Blend until smooth
3. Serve chilled and enjoy!

Nutrition Info: Calories: 145; Fat: 4g; Carbohydrates: 1.6g; Protein: 0.6g

Creamy Peachy Shake

Servings: 2
Cooking Time: 5 Minutes
Ingredients:
- 2 scoops vanilla protein powder
- 2 cups peaches
- ¼ cup fat-free Greek yogurt
- ½ cup orange juice

Directions:
1. Add all the ingredients except vegetables/fruits first
2. Blend until smooth
3. Add the vegetable/fruits
4. Blend until smooth
5. Add a few ice cubes and serve the smoothie
6. Enjoy!

Nutrition Info: Calories: 380; Fat: 3g; Carbohydrates: 72g; Protein: 20g

The Cacao Super Smoothie

Servings: 1
Cooking Time: 10 Minutes
Ingredients:
- ½ avocado, peeled, pitted, sliced
- ½ cup frozen blueberries, unsweetened
- ½ cup almond milk, vanilla, unsweetened
- ½ cup half and half
- 1 scoop whey vanilla protein powder
- 1 tablespoon cacao powder
- Liquid stevia

Directions:
1. Add listed ingredients to a blender
2. Blend until you get a smooth and creamy texture
3. Serve chilled and enjoy!

Nutrition Info: Calories: 445; Fat: 14g; Carbohydrates: 9g; Protein: 16g

Green Protein Smoothie

Servings: 2
Cooking Time: 10 Minutes
Ingredients:
- 2 bananas
- 4 cups mixed greens
- 2 tablespoons almond butter
- 1 cup almond milk, unsweetened

Directions:
1. Add all the listed ingredients to a blender
2. Blend until you have a smooth and creamy texture
3. Serve chilled and enjoy!

Nutrition Info: Calories: 230; Fat: 5.8g; Carbohydrates: 39.5g; Protein: 7.8g

Berry Orange Madness

Servings: 2-3
Cooking Time: 2 Minutes
Ingredients:
- 1 cup mixed berries (fresh or frozen)
- 1 large orange, peeled, seeded and segmented
- 1 cup low fat plain yogurt
- 1 banana, chopped (frozen)
- ¼ teaspoon vanilla extract
- 1-2 ice cubes

Directions:
1. Pour all the ingredients into your blender and process until smooth.

Nutrition Info: (Per Serving): Calories-210, Fat-2 g, Protein- 8.3 g, Carbohydrates- 40 g

Strawberry Coconut Snowflake

Servings: 2
Cooking Time: 2 Minutes
Ingredients:
- ½ unsweetened, fresh coconut milk
- 1 cup whole strawberries (fresh or frozen)
- ½ cup plain low fat Greek yogurt
- ¼ cup freshly squeezed orange
- ½ teaspoon raw organic honey
- 2-3 ice cubes

Directions:
1. Just place all the ingredients into the blender and pulse until smooth. Serve immediately!

Nutrition Info: (Per Serving): Calories- 160, Fat- 2.8 g, Protein- 12 g, Carbohydrates- 24 g

WEIGHT LOSS SMOOTHIES

Blueberry–avocado Smoothie

Servings: 1
Cooking Time: 2 Minutes
Ingredients:
- ½ cup blueberries (fresh or frozen)
- 3 tablespoons ripe avocado flesh
- 1 tablespoon Chia seeds, soaked for 10 minutes
- 1 teaspoon pure coconut oil
- ½ tablespoon raw organic honey
- A large pinch of cinnamon powder
- 1 cup filtered water

Directions:
1. Place all the above listed ingredients into your blender and pulse until smooth.

Nutrition Info: (Per Serving): Calories-330, Fat- 25 g, Protein- 4 g, Carbohydrates- 30 g

Kale Celery Smoothie

Servings: 2
Cooking Time: 10 Minutes
Ingredients:
- 3 cups kale, chopped
- 2 stalks celery, diced
- 1 red apple, cored and diced
- 2 cups almond milk, unsweetened
- 1 ¼ cups ice
- 2 teaspoons honey
- 2 tablespoons flaxseed, ground

Directions:
1. Add all the listed ingredients to a blender
2. Blend until you have a smooth and creamy texture
3. Serve chilled and enjoy!

Nutrition Info: Calories: 341; Fat: 29.8g; Carbohydrates: 18.6g; Protein: 5.3g

Peanut Butter Berry Smoothie

Servings: 2
Cooking Time: 2 Minutes
Ingredients:
- 1 tablespoon peanut butter
- 2 cups strawberry (fresh or frozen)
- 1 large banana, chopped (fresh or frozen)
- ½ cup plain or Greek yogurt
- A handful of ice cubes

Directions:
1. Add all the ingredients into the blender and whip it up until smooth and nice.

2. Pour into cool serving glasses and enjoy.
Nutrition Info: (Per Serving): Calories- 327, Fat- 7 g, Protein- 18 g, Carbohydrates- 55 g

Tropical Avocado Smoothie

Servings: 3
Cooking Time: 5 Minutes
Ingredients:
- 1 ½ cups whole strawberries (fresh r frozen)
- ¾ cup organic coconut milk
- 1 ½ cup mango, chopped
- 1 ½ cups freshly squeezed pineapple juice
- 1/3 cup avocado, chopped
- 2 kiwi fruits, peeled and chopped

Directions:
1. Place all the ingredients into your blender and run it on high for 20 seconds or until done.
Nutrition Info: (Per Serving): Calories- 185, Fat- 6 g, Protein- 2.2 g, Carbohydrates- 33 g

Straight Up Avocado And Kale Smoothie

Servings: 2
Cooking Time: 5 Minutes
Ingredients:
- 1 tablespoon spirulina
- 1 cup chamomile tea
- 1 tablespoon Chia seeds
- 1 stalk celery
- 1 cup cucumber
- ½ avocado, diced
- 1 cup kale, chopped

Directions:
1. Add all the ingredients except vegetables/fruits first
2. Blend until smooth
3. Add the vegetable/fruits
4. Blend until smooth
5. Add a few ice cubes and serve the smoothie
6. Enjoy!
Nutrition Info: Calories: 236; Fat: 6g; Carbohydrates: 46g; Protein: 4g

Meanie-greenie Weigh Loss Smoothie

Servings: 2-3
Cooking Time: 5 Minutes
Ingredients:
- 1 cup kale, stems removed
- 1 cup green cucumber, de-seeded and chopped
- 1 celery stalk, chopped

- 1 small pear, peeled, cored and chopped
- 1 teaspoon freshly grated ginger
- A handful of parsley
- 1 ½ cups of filtered water
- 1 teaspoon freshly squeezed lemon juice

Directions:

1. Place all the ingredients in the order listed above and pulse until the desired consistency is attained.

Nutrition Info: (Per Serving): Calories- 64.3, Fat- 0.3 g, Protein- 1 g, Carbohydrates- 15.8 g

Peanut Butter, Banana And Cacao Smoothie

Servings: 2
Cooking Time: 5 Minutes
Ingredients:

- 1 cup unsweetened almond milk
- 2 tablespoons peanut butter
- 2 large ripe bananas (fresh or frozen)
- 2 teaspoons cacao powder
- ½ teaspoon vanilla extract
- 1 teaspoon raw organic honey
- 3-4 cubes of ice

Directions:

1. Add all the ingredients in the blender and process until smooth.

Nutrition Info: (Per Serving): Calories- 345, Fat- 16 g, Protein- 11 g, Carbohydrates- 90 g

Banana-blackberry Smoothie

Servings: 2
Cooking Time: 5 Minutes
Ingredients:

- 1 cup unsweetened almond milk
- 1 apple, cored and chopped
- 1 cup blackberries (fresh or frozen)
- 1 banana, chopped (fresh or frozen)
- ½ cup plain yogurt
- ½ teaspoon vanilla extract
- 3 medjool dates, pitted
- 2 teaspoons flaxseed powder
- 1 teaspoon cinnamon powder

Directions:

1. Place everything into your blender and whizz up for 30 seconds until smoothie is well combined without lumps.

Nutrition Info: (Per Serving): Calories- 218, Fat- 3.5 g, Protein- 8.9 g, Carbohydrates- 43 g

Clemintine Dreamsicle Smoothie

Servings: 1
Cooking Time: 2 Minutes
Ingredients:
- 4 Clementine, peeled and chopped
- 1 small banana (fresh or frozen)
- ¼ cup unsweetened almond milk
- ½ teaspoon raw organic honey
- ½ teaspoon vanilla extract
- A pinch of turmeric powder
- A pinch of Celtic salt
- 3-4 ice cubes

Directions:
1. Place the ingredients listed above into your high speed blender and process until the smoothie is thick and creamy.

Nutrition Info: (Per Serving): Calories- 145, Fat- 0.3 g, Protein- 6.6 g, Carbohydrates- 33.5 g

Healthy Raspberry And Coconut Glass

Servings: 1
Cooking Time: 10 Minutes
Ingredients:
- ¼ cup raspberries
- 1 tablespoon pepitas
- 1 tablespoon coconut oil
- ½ cup of coconut milk
- 1 cup 50/50 salad mix
- 1 ½ cups of water
- 1 pack stevia

Directions:
1. Add listed ingredients to a blender
2. Blend until you have a smooth and creamy texture
3. Serve chilled and enjoy!

Nutrition Info: Calories: 408; Fat: 41g; Carbohydrates: 10g; Protein: 5g

Banana And Spinach Raspberry Smoothie

Servings: 2
Cooking Time: 5 Minutes
Ingredients:
- 1 tablespoons cilantro
- 1 cup crushed ice
- 1 tablespoon ground flaxseed
- ½ cup raspberries
- 2 dates
- 2 bananas

- 1 cup spinach, chopped

Directions:
1. Add all the ingredients except vegetables/fruits first
2. Blend until smooth
3. Add the vegetable/fruits
4. Blend until smooth
5. Add a few ice cubes and serve the smoothie
6. Enjoy!

Nutrition Info: Calories: 120; Fat: 2g; Carbohydrates: 30g; Protein: 3g

Raspberry- Grapefruit Smoothie

Servings: 2-3
Cooking Time: 5 Minutes
Ingredients:
- 2 cups fresh spinach, chopped
- ½ grapefruits, peeled and de seeded
- ½ cup raspberries (fresh or frozen)
- 1 California orange, peeled and de seeded
- ¼ cup whole strawberries (fresh or frozen)
- 1 tablespoon Chia seeds, soaked
- 1 ½ cups of filtered water

Directions:
1. To your blender, add all the items listed above and blend until smooth and creamy.

Nutrition Info: (Per Serving): Calories- 164, Fat- 5.5 g, Protein- 5.6 g, Carbohydrates- 29 g

Chia-blueberry Smoothie

Servings: 2
Cooking Time: 5 Minutes
Ingredients:
- ½ cup blueberries, (fresh or frozen)
- 6 ounces of plain or Greek yogurt
- ½ banana, chopped
- 1 tablespoons Chia seeds, soaked
- A pinch of cinnamon powder
- 4 ounces of filtered water

Directions:
1. Add all the ingredients into the blender jar and pulse it on high for 30 seconds or until smooth.

Nutrition Info: (Per Serving): Calories- 325, Fat- 20 g, Protein-8 g, Carbohydrates-32 g

Kale Strawberry Smoothie

Servings: 2
Cooking Time: 10 Minutes
Ingredients:

- 2 cups kale, chopped
- 2 bananas
- 2 cups strawberries
- 2 cups ice
- 2 cups yogurt

Directions:
1. Add all the listed ingredients to a blender
2. Blend until you have a smooth and creamy texture
3. Serve chilled and enjoy!

Nutrition Info: Calories: 358; Fat: 3.8g; Carbohydrates: 62.3g; Protein: 18.2g

KID FRIENDLY HEALTHY SMOOTHIES

Pina- Banana Quickie

Servings: 2
Cooking Time: 5 Minutes
Ingredients:
- 1 cup plain unsweetened soy milk or almond milk
- 1 small ripe banana, chopped (fresh or frozen)
- 1 cup pineapple, peeled and chopped
- 1 teaspoon flaxseeds
- 3-4 ice cubes

Directions:
1. Add all the ingredients into the high speed blender and whizz until smooth.

Nutrition Info: (Per Serving): Calories- 213, Fat- 4.8 g, Protein- 8 g, Carbohydrates- 35 g

Pineapple Papaya Perfection Smoothie

Servings: 3
Cooking Time: 5 Minutes
Ingredients:
- 2 cups papaya. Peeled and chopped
- 1 cup plain low fat yogurt
- ½ cup pineapple, peeled and chopped
- 1 teaspoon grated coconut
- 1 teaspoon flax seed powder
- 2 teaspoon freshly squeezed lemon juice
- 4-5 ice cubes

Directions:
1. To make this smoothie, place everything into the blender and pulse until smooth. Serve immediately.

Nutrition Info: (Per Serving): Calories- 230, Fat- 1.4 g, Protein- 12.5 g, Carbohydrates- 65 g

Raw Chocolate Smoothie

Servings: 2
Cooking Time: 10 Minutes
Ingredients:
- 2 medium bananas
- 4 tablespoons peanut butter, raw
- 1 cup almond milk
- 3 tablespoons cocoa powder, raw
- 2 tablespoons honey, raw

Directions:
1. Add all the listed ingredients to a blender
2. Blend until you have a smooth and creamy texture
3. Serve chilled and enjoy!

Nutrition Info: Calories: 217; Fat: 2.8g; Carbohydrates: 52.7g; Protein: 3.4g

The Strawberry Almond Smoothie

Servings: 1
Cooking Time: 10 Minutes
Ingredients:
- 16 ounces unsweetened almond milk, vanilla
- 1 pack stevia
- 4 ounces heavy cream
- 1 scoop vanilla whey protein
- ¼ cup frozen strawberries, unsweetened

Directions:
1. Add all the ingredients except vegetables/fruits first
2. Blend until smooth
3. Add the vegetable/fruits
4. Blend until smooth
5. Add a few ice cubes and serve the smoothie
6. Enjoy!

Nutrition Info: Calories: 465; Fat: 28g; Carbohydrates: 57g; Protein: 6g

Peanut Butter Broccoli Smoothie

Servings: 3
Cooking Time: 5 Minutes
Ingredients:
- 1 cup unsweetened almond milk
- 1 cup fresh spinach, washed and chopped
- 1 cup broccoli florets, washed and chopped
- 1 large kale leaf, washed and chopped
- 1 ripe banana, chopped
- 2 teaspoons peanut butter
- 1 teaspoon raw organic honey (optional)

Directions:
1. Add all the ingredients into the high speed blender and whizz until smooth.

Nutrition Info: (Per Serving): Calories- 325, Fat- 14 g, Protein- 10 g, Carbohydrates- 46 g

Delish Pineapple And Coconut Milk Smoothie

Servings: 2
Cooking Time: 5 Minutes
Ingredients:
- ¾ cup of coconut water
- ¼ cup pineapple, frozen

Directions:
1. Add listed ingredients to a blender
2. Blend on high until you have a smooth and creamy texture
3. Serve chilled and enjoy!

Nutrition Info: Calories: 132; Fat: 12g; Carbohydrates: 7g; Protein: 1g

Pineapple Banana Smoothie

Servings: 2
Cooking Time: 10 Minutes
Ingredients:
- 2 apples
- 4 cups spinach
- 2 bananas
- 2 cups pineapples
- 2 cups of water

Directions:
1. Add all the listed ingredients to a blender
2. Blend until you have a smooth and creamy texture
3. Serve chilled and enjoy!

Nutrition Info: Calories: 317; Fat: 1.2g; Carbohydrates: 81.6g; Protein: 4.5g

Apple Berry Smoothie

Servings: 2
Cooking Time: 10 Minutes
Ingredients:
- 2 large apples
- 4 cups spinach
- 2 cups berries, mixed
- 2 cups of water

Directions:
1. Add all the listed ingredients to a blender
2. Blend until you have a smooth and creamy texture
3. Serve chilled and enjoy!

Nutrition Info: Calories: 210; Fat: 1.1g; Carbohydrates: 50g; Protein: 3.3g

Cool Coco-loco Cream Shake

Servings: 1
Cooking Time: 10 Minutes
Ingredients:
- ½ cup coconut milk
- 2 tablespoons Dutch-processed cocoa powder, unsweetened
- 1 cup brewed coffee, chilled
- 1-2 packs stevia
- 1 tablespoon hemp seeds

Directions:
1. Add all the ingredients except vegetables/fruits first
2. Blend until smooth
3. Add the vegetable/fruits

4. Blend until smooth
5. Add a few ice cubes and serve the smoothie
6. Enjoy!
Nutrition Info: Calories: 337; Fat: 11g; Carbohydrates: 38g; Protein: 1g

Delicious Creamy Choco Shake

Servings: 1
Cooking Time: 10 Minutes
Ingredients:
- ½ cup heavy cream
- 2 tablespoons cocoa powder
- 1 pack stevia
- 1 cup water

Directions:
1. Add all the ingredients except vegetables/fruits first
2. Blend until smooth
3. Add the vegetable/fruits
4. Blend until smooth
5. Add a few ice cubes and serve the smoothie
6. Enjoy!
Nutrition Info: Calories: 180; Fat: 6g; Carbohydrates: 30g; Protein: 3g

Grape- Lettuce Chiller

Servings: 2
Cooking Time: 2 Minutes
Ingredients:
- 1 cup green grapes, seedless
- 1 large cup romaine lettuce, washed and chopped
- ½ large apple, cored and chopped
- 2-3 teaspoons freshly squeezed lemon juice
- ½ teaspoon raw organic honey
- 4-5 ice cubes

Directions:
1. To you blender, add the above ingredient and pulse until smooth.
Nutrition Info: (Per Serving): Calories-82, Fat- 0 g, Protein- 1.4 g , Carbohydrates- 22 g

Coconut Strawberry Punch

Servings: 2
Cooking Time: 5 Minutes
Ingredients:
- 1 cup fresh coconut water
- 8 – 10 whole strawberries (fresh or frozen)
- ½ cup plain yogurt
- 1 tablespoon freshly squeezed lemon juice

- 2-3 ice cubes

Directions:
1. Place all the ingredients into the blender and puree until everything is well combined.

Nutrition Info: (Per Serving): Calories- 400, Fat- 3 g, Protein- 4 g, Carbohydrates- 10 g

Chocolate Spinach Smoothie

Servings: 4
Cooking Time: 10 Minutes

Ingredients:
- 4 cups banana, sliced
- 2 cups spinach, packed
- 6 tablespoons peanut butter
- 2 cups almond milk
- ½ cup of cocoa powder
- 2 tablespoons flaxseeds, grounded

Directions:
1. Add all the listed ingredients to a blender
2. Blend until you have a smooth and creamy texture
3. Serve chilled and enjoy!

Nutrition Info: Calories: 356; Fat: 16.2g; Carbohydrates: 51.7g; Protein: 13g

Peanut Butter Jelly Smoothie

Servings: 2
Cooking Time: 2 Minutes

Ingredients:
- 1 cup whole raspberries (fresh or frozen)
- 2 teaspoons peanut butter
- ½ large banana, chopped
- 1 cup unsweetened almond milk
- ½ teaspoon raw organic honey
- 2-3 ice cubes

Directions:
1. Pour all the ingredients into your blender and process until smooth.

Nutrition Info: (Per Serving): Calories-270, Fat- 12 g, Protein- 7 g, Carbohydrates- 40 g

HEART HEALTHY SMOOTHIES

Banana-beet Smoothie

Servings: 2
Cooking Time: 5 Minutes
Ingredients:
- 1 cup whole strawberries (fresh or frozen)
- 1 large red beet, peeled and chipped
- 1 large banana (fresh or frozen)
- 1 orange, peeled and de seeded
- 2 cups fresh spinach
- 1 cup fresh kale, stems removed
- 1 cup unsweetened almond milk

Directions:
1. Add everything to the blender jar, secure the lid and pulse until thick and creamy.

Nutrition Info: (Per Serving): Calories- 333, Fat- 4 g, Protein- 10 g, Carbohydrates- 71 g

Peach And Celery Smoothie

Servings: 2
Cooking Time: 5 Minutes
Ingredients:
- ½ green cucumber, chopped with peel on
- 1 large peach, pitted and chopped
- 1 orange, peeled and de seeded
- 2 tablespoons avocado flesh
- 2-3 stalks celery, washed and chopped
- 2 cups fresh Swiss chard, chopped
- ¾ cup filtered water
- 3-4 cubes of ice

Directions:
1. Combine all the above ingredients in your blender and process until the desired consistency is obtained.

Nutrition Info: (Per Serving): Calories- 255, Fat- 0 g, Protein- 8 g, Carbohydrates- 50 g

Almond- Citrus Punch

Servings: 2
Cooking Time: 2 Minutes
Ingredients:
- 1 cup unsweetened almond milk
- ½ cup freshly squeezed orange juice
- 1 tablespoon raw organic honey
- 1/3 cup freshly squeezed lime juice
- 1 tablespoon freshly squeezed lemon
- ¼ teaspoon vanilla extract
- A handful of ice cubes

Directions:
1.   Pour all the ingredients into the blender and blend for 45 seconds until well combined.
Nutrition Info: (Per Serving): Calories- 150, Fat- 4 g, Protein- 2 g, Carbohydrates- 30 g

Spinach And Grape Smoothie

Servings: 1 Large
Cooking Time: 5 Minutes
Ingredients:
- 1 cup red grapes (seedless)
- 2 cups baby spinach
- 1 banana (fresh or frozen)
- 1 tablespoon Chia seeds (soaked)
- 1 teaspoon freshly squeezed lemon juice
- A handful of ice cubes

Directions:
1.   Load all the ingredients into your blender jar and secure it tightly with a lid.
2.   Pulse it on medium speed for 30 seconds and on high for 1 minute or until smooth.
Nutrition Info: (Per Serving): Calories-107, Fat-2.4 g, Protein-1.5 g, Carbohydrates-26.5 g

Strawberry-chia Smoothie

Servings: 2
Cooking Time: 2 Minutes
Ingredients:
- 1 ½ cups whole strawberries (fresh or frozen)
- 2 medium bananas, fresh or frozen
- 1 cup unsweetened almond milk
- 2 tablespoon Chia seeds, soaked
- 3-4 fresh collard leaves, stems removed
- 2-3 ice cubes (optional)

Directions:
1.   Add all the ingredients into your blender and whip it up until the smoothie is thick and frothy.
Nutrition Info: (Per Serving): Calories- 340, Fat- 0 g, Protein- 10 g, Carbohydrates- 65 g

Chia-cacao Melon Smoothie

Servings: 2
Cooking Time: 5 Minutes
Ingredients:
- 1 cup fresh strawberries
- 1 cup cantaloupe, chopped
- 1 large banana (fresh or frozen)
- 2 large chard leaves, chopped
- 1 cup unsweetened almond milk

- 1 tablespoon cacao powder
- 1 tablespoons Chia seeds, soaked

Directions:
1. Pour all the ingredients into your blender and whizz it up on high speed for 45 seconds or until done.

Nutrition Info: (Per Serving): Calories- 330, Fat- 0 g, Protein- 11 g, Carbohydrates- 62 g

Hemp-avocado Smoothie

Servings: 2
Cooking Time: 5 Minutes
Ingredients:
- A red apple, cored and chopped
- 1 tablespoon avocado flesh
- 1 cup unsweetened almond milk
- 2 tablespoon hemp seeds
- 2 cups fresh baby spinach

Directions:
1. Pour all the ingredients into your blender and run in on high for 1 minute. Pour into tall glasses and enjoy!

Nutrition Info: (Per Serving): Calories- 350, Fat- 0 g, Protein- 10 g, Carbohydrates- 43 g

Pineapple-pear And Spinach Smoothie

Servings: 2
Cooking Time: 5 Minutes
Ingredients:
- 1 cup pineapple, peeled and chopped
- ½ green pear, cored and chopped
- ¾ cup unsweetened almond milk
- 2 cups baby spinach
- 1 cup fresh kale
- 2 tablespoons Chia seeds, soaked
- ¼ teaspoon freshly grated ginger
- 1 teaspoon freshly squeezed lemon juice

Directions:
1. First add the fruits to your blender and whizz for 30 seconds until pureed.
2. Then add the rest f the ingredients and pulse for 1 minute or until a creamy smoothie is got.
3. Pour into tall glasses and enjoy!

Nutrition Info: (Per Serving): Caloris-340, Fat- 0 g, Protein- 8 g, Carbohydrates- 47 g

Ginger Banana Kick

Servings: 2
Cooking Time: 5 Minutes
Ingredients:
- 1 large banana, chopped (fresh or frozen)
- 1 large orange, peeled and de seeded

- 2 cups almond milk or plain soy milk
- 1 teaspoon freshly grated ginger
- ¼ teaspoon vanilla extract
- ½ teaspoon raw, organic honey (optional)
- 1 few ice cubes

Directions:

1. Load your blender jar with the ingredients listed above and puree it until nice and thick.

Nutrition Info: (Per Serving): Calories- 181, Fat- 5.1 g, Proteins- 8.3 g, Carbohydrates- 30 g

Mint And Avocado Smoothie

Servings: 3
Cooking Time: 5 Minutes

Ingredients:

- 2 cups unsweetened almond milk
- 1 medium banana, chopped
- 2 cups of fresh spinach
- 1 kiwi, peeled and quartered
- Freshly squeezed juice of 1 lime
- 6-8 fresh mint leaves
- ½ avocado, pitted and chopped
- 1 teaspoon freshly grated ginger

Directions:

1. Place all the above listed ingredients in the same order into your blender jar and process it until thick and smooth.

Nutrition Info: (Per Serving): Calories- 254, Fat- 12 g, Protein-10 g, Carbohydrates- 31 g

Mango-ginger Tango

Servings: 2
Cooking Time: 5 Minutes

Ingredients:

- 1 cup pineapple, peeled and chopped
- 1 cup mango, chopped
- 1 large orange, peeled and de seeded
- ½ cup filtered water
- 2 cups fresh kale, stems removed and chopped
- 1 teaspoon freshly grated ginger
- 2-3 cubes of ice

Directions:

1. Place all the ingredients into the blended one by one and pulse until smooth.

Nutrition Info: (Per Serving): Calories- 355, Fat- 0 g, Protein- 9 g, Carbohydrates- 88 g

Vanilla- Mango Madness

Servings: 1
Cooking Time: 2 Minutes

Ingredients:

- 1 cup mango, chopped (fresh or frozen)

- 1 cup plain yogurt
- 1 tablespoon freshly squeezed lemon juice
- ¼ teaspoon vanilla extract
- ¼ teaspoon nutmeg powder
- 1 teaspoon raw organic honey
- A pinch of Celtic salt
- ¼ cup filtered water

Directions:
1. To your blender jar, add all the ingredients and whizz until thick and creamy.

Nutrition Info: (Per Serving): Calories- 160, Fat- 2 g, Protein- 7 g, Carbohydrates- 29.3 g

Peach-ban-illa Smoothie

Servings: 2 Small
Cooking Time: 5 Minutes
Ingredients:
- 1 ¼ cup peaches, pitted and chopped
- 1 large banana (fresh or frozen)
- 1 cup plain yogurt
- 1 teaspoon vanilla extract
- 1 teaspoon Chia seeds, soaked
- A handful of ice

Directions:
1. Combine all the ingredients in the blender and blend until the desired consistency is got.

Nutrition Info: (Per Serving): Calories- 170, Fat- 2 g, Protein- 5 g, Carbohydrates- 45 g

Oats And Berry Smoothie

Servings: 1
Cooking Time: 2 Minutes
Ingredients:
- 1 small ripe banana (fresh or frozen)
- 1 cup whole strawberries (fresh or frozen)
- ¼ cup almonds (soaked and de-skinned)
- ½ cup rolled oats
- 1 teaspoon raw organic honey
- 1/3 cup plain yogurt
- ¼ teaspoon vanilla extract

Directions:
1. Load the blender jar with all the above listed ingredients and process it for a minute until thick and creamy.
2. Pour into a glass and serve immediately!

Nutrition Info: (Per Serving): Calories- 450, Fat- 15.7 g, Protein- 17.5 g, Carbohydrates- 74 g

OVERALL HEALTH AND WELLNESS SMOOTHIES

Apple Cucumber

Servings: 2-3
Cooking Time: 5 Minutes
Ingredients:
- 1 green apple, cored and chopped
- 1 green cucumber, deseeded and chopped
- 1/3 cup collard greens, chopped
- 1 ½ teaspoons Chia seeds, soaked
- 1 tablespoon freshly squeezed lemon juice
- 5-6 fresh mint leaves
- 1 cup filtered water
- 3-4 ice cubes

Directions:
1. Add all the above ingredients into your blender jar and pulse until thick and frothy.

Nutrition Info: (Per Serving): Calories- 114, Fat- 3.2 g, Protein- 3.1 g, Carbohydrates- 25 g

Dragon- Berry Smoothie

Servings: 3
Cooking Time: 5 Minutes
Ingredients:
- ½ cup dragon fruits, peeled and chopped
- ½ cup raspberries (fresh or frozen)
- ½ cup spinach, chopped and washed
- ½ cup mixed greens, washed and chopped
- 1 ripe banana, chopped
- 1-2 dates, pitted
- 1 ½ cups homemade almond milk
- A pinch of cinnamon powder

Directions:
1. To your high speed blender, add all the above mentioned items and process on high for 30 seconds. Pour into serving glasses and enjoy immediately.

Nutrition Info: (Per Serving): Calories- 320, Fat-7.4 g, Protein- 5 g, Carbohydrates- 62 g

Blue Dragon Smoothie

Servings: 2
Cooking Time: 5 Minutes
Ingredients:
- ½ cup unsweetened almond milk
- ½ cup dragon fruits, peeled and chopped
- A handful of blueberries (fresh or frozen)
- A handful of fresh kale
- A handful of baby spinach
- 1 tablespoon Chia seeds, soaked

- 3-4 ice cubes

Directions:
1. Add all the above ingredients into your blender jar and pulse until thick and frothy.

Nutrition Info: (Per Serving): Calories- 135, Fat- 2.3 g, Protein- 4.8 g, Carbohydrates- 22g

Finana Smoothie

Servings: 2
Cooking Time: 5 Minutes
Ingredients:
- 1 banana, chopped (fresh or frozen)
- 2 figs, chopped
- A handful of mixed greens, washed
- ½ cup filtered water
- 1 teaspoon raw organic honey
- 2-3 ice cubes

Directions:
1. Load your blender with all the ingredients and puree until smoothie is thick and creamy.

Nutrition Info: (Per Serving): Calories- 330, Fat- 1.7 g, Protein- 5.5 g, Carbohydrates- 87 g

Cinnaberry Green Smoothie

Servings: 3
Cooking Time: 5 Minutes
Ingredients:
- 2 cups unsweetened almond milk
- A handful of baby spinach, washed
- ½ cup mixed greens
- 2 small ripe bananas, sliced (fresh or frozen)
- ½ cup whole raspberries (fresh or frozen)
- 5 teaspoons cacao powder
- 1/3 teaspoon cinnamon powder
- 3-4 ice cubes

Directions:
1. To your high speed bender, add all the ingredients and process until smooth.

Nutrition Info: (Per Serving): Calories- 375, Fat- 15 g, Protein- 19 g, Carbohydrates- 55 g

Drink Your Salad Smoothie

Servings: 2
Cooking Time: 5 Minutes
Ingredients:
- 4 vine tomatoes, washed
- 1 teaspoon avocado flesh
- 1 red bell pepper, deseeded
- ½ green zucchini, chopped

- 3-4 celery stalks, chopped
- ¼ white onion
- 1 teaspoon of flax seed powder
- A pinch of cayenne pepper
- A pinch of paprika or chili powder
- ¼ cup filtered water

Directions:
1. Dump all the ingredients into the blender and whip it up until the smoothie is thick and creamy.

Nutrition Info: (Per Serving): Calories-458, Fat- 16.5 g, Protein- 16.8 g, Carbohydrates- 78 g

Lychee Green Smoothie

Servings: 2
Cooking Time: 2 Minutes
Ingredients:
- 1/3 cup baby spinach
- ½ cup cantaloupe, peeled and chopped
- ½ cup grapes, deseeded
- 3-4 lychees, peeled and pitted
- 1 cup filtered water
- 1 teaspoon freshly squeezed lemon juice
- ½ teaspoon freshly grated ginger
- 3-4 ice cubes

Directions:
1. Just place all the ingredients into the blender and pulse until smooth. Serve immediately!

Nutrition Info: (Per Serving): Calories- 77, Fat- 0.7 g, Protein- 1.9 g, Carbohydrates- 20 g

Red Healing Potion

Servings: 3
Cooking Time: 5 Minutes
Ingredients:
- 2 cups fresh coconut water
- 1 ½ cup pomegranate seeds
- 1 ¼ cup of red grapes, deseeded
- 1 cup whole strawberries (fresh or frozen)
- 2 tablespoons freshly squeezed lemon juice
- 4-5 ice cubes

Directions:
1. Place everything in your blender jar and whizz until smooth and frothy.

Nutrition Info: (Per Serving): Calories- 182, Fat-1.2 g, Protein- 4.3 g, Carbohydrates- 44 g

Water-mato Green Smoothie

Servings: 2
Cooking Time: 2 Minutes
Ingredients:
- 1 cup watermelon, chopped (seedless)

- ½ cup whole strawberries (fresh or frozen)
- 1 cup mixed greens, washed and chopped
- ¼ cup vine tomatoes
- 2 teaspoon freshly squeezed lemon juice
- ¼ cup filtered water
- 2-3 ice cubes

Directions:
1. Whizz up all the above listed ingredients in your blender for 20 seconds and serve. Enjoy immediately.

Nutrition Info: (Per Serving): Calories- 160, Fat- 0.7 g, Protein- 4.5 g, Carbohydrates- 27 g

Crunchy Mango Squash Smoothie

Servings: 2
Cooking Time: 2 Minutes
Ingredients:
- ½ cup squash, peeled and chopped
- ½ cup mango, peeled and chopped
- 1 large orange, peeled and deseeded
- 1 cup filtered water
- 2 teaspoons chopped walnuts
- ½ teaspoon cinnamon powder
- 5-6 ice cubes

Directions:
1. Add all the above ingredients into your blender jar and pulse until thick and frothy.

Nutrition Info: (Per Serving): Calories- 150, Fat- 7.2 g, Protein- 4.2 g, Carbohydrates- 23 g

Nutty Apple Smoothie

Servings: 2
Cooking Time: 2 Minutes
Ingredients:
- 2 apple, cored and chopped
- 2/3 cup plain low fat yogurt
- ¼ cup toasted peanuts
- 3 teaspoons raw organic honey
- 1 teaspoon almond butter
- 3-4 ice cubes

Directions:
1. Pour all the ingredients into your blender and process until smooth.

Nutrition Info: (Per Serving): Calories- 291, Fat- 11g, Protein- 8.3 g, Carbohydrates- 48 g

Pear-simmon Smoothie

Servings: 4
Cooking Time: 5 Minutes
Ingredients:
- 4 persimmons, chopped
- 2 small apples, cored and chopped

- 2 small pears, cored and chopped
- 2 handfuls of baby spinach
- 2 cups of mixed greens
- 1 cup filtered water
- 2 teaspoons of freshly squeezed lemon juice
- 4-5 ice cubes

Directions:
1. Place all the above ingredients into the blender jar and process until the mixture is thick and creamy.

Nutrition Info: (Per Serving): Calories- 239, Fat- 1 g, Protein- 3 g, Carbohydrates- 63 g

Citrus Coconut Punch

Servings: 2-3
Cooking Time: 5 Minutes
Ingredients:
- 1 yellow grapefruit, peeled and deseeded
- 2 mandarins, peeled and deseeded
- 1 large lime, peeled and deseeded
- Freshly squeezed juice of 1 lemon
- 2 cups fresh coconut water
- 1 teaspoon freshly grated ginger
- 4-5 ice cubes

Directions:
1. Load all the ingredients into your blender and whizz until smooth.

Nutrition Info: (Per Serving): Calories- 211, Fat- 0.6 g, Protein- 4.2 g, Carbohydrates- 53 g

Fig Berry Dragon Smoothie

Servings: 4 -5
Cooking Time: 5 Minutes
Ingredients:
- 1 cup dragon fruits, peeled and chopped
- 4 figs, chopped
- ½ cup blackberries (fresh or frozen)
- ½ cup raspberries (fresh or frozen)
- 2 cups mixed greens
- 2 handfuls of baby spinach
- 1 cup freshly prepared pomegranate juice
- 4-5 ice cubes

Directions:
1. Add all the above ingredients into your blender jar and pulse until thick and frothy.

Nutrition Info: (Per Serving): Calories- 245, Fat- 3.2 g, Protein-6.2 g, Carbohydrates- 56 g

LOW FAT SMOOTHIES

Mini Pepper Popper Smoothie

Servings: 2
Cooking Time: 5 Minutes
Ingredients:
- 5 ounces mini peppers, seeded
- 4 ounces pineapple
- 1 orange, peeled
- 3 tablespoons almonds
- ½ lemon, juiced
- 1 cup of water
- 1 teaspoon rose hip powder

Directions:
1. Add all the listed ingredients to a blender
2. Blend until you have a smooth and creamy texture
3. Serve chilled and enjoy!

Nutrition Info: Calories: 190; Fat: 8g; Carbohydrates: 21g; Protein: 5g

Pomegranate- Ginger Melba

Servings: 3
Cooking Time: 2 Minutes
Ingredients:
- 2 cups freshly prepared pomegranate juice
- 2 bananas, chopped (fresh or frozen)
- 1 cup low fat plain Greek yogurt
- 1 teaspoon freshly grated ginger
- 5-6 ice cubes

Directions:
1. Place all the ingredients into your blender and run it on medium high speed for 1-2 minutes or until done.

Nutrition Info: (Per Serving): Calories- 195, Fat- 2.2 g, Protein- 8 g, Carbohydrates- 40 g

Low Fat Tropical Pleasure

Servings: 4
Cooking Time: 5 Minutes
Ingredients:
- 1 cup banana, chopped (fresh or frozen)
- 1 cup mango, chopped (fresh or frozen)
- 1 cup kiwi, peeled and chopped (fresh or frozen)
- 1 cup pineapple, chopped (fresh or frozen)
- ½ cup freshly squeezed orange juice
- 1 cup low fat buttermilk
- 4-5 ice cubes

Directions:

1. Place all the ingredients into the high speed blender jar and run it on high for 20 seconds until everything is well combined. Pour into serving glass and enjoy!
Nutrition Info: (Per Serving): Calories-220, Fat- 14 g, Protein- 4 g, Carbohydrates- 48 g

The Summer Hearty Shake

Servings: 2
Cooking Time: 5 Minutes
Ingredients:
- 1 cup frozen blackberries
- ¾ cup whole milk vanilla yogurt
- ½ cup unsweetened vanilla almond milk
- ½ cup frozen strawberries
- ½ cup frozen peaches
- 1 tablespoon hemp seeds
- Dash of ground cinnamon

Directions:
1. Add all the ingredients except vegetables/fruits first
2. Blend until smooth
3. Add the vegetable/fruits
4. Blend until smooth
5. Add a few ice cubes and serve the smoothie
6. Enjoy!

Nutrition Info: Calories: 187; Fat: 6g; Carbohydrates: 23g; Protein: 6g

Papaya, Lemon And Cayenne Pepper Smoothie

Servings: 2
Cooking Time: 5 Minutes
Ingredients:
- 2 cups papaya
- ½ teaspoon cayenne pepper
- 3 tablespoons lemon juice

Directions:
1. Add all the listed ingredients to a blender
2. Blend until you have a smooth and creamy texture
3. Serve chilled and enjoy!

Nutrition Info: Calories: 121; Fat: 6g; Carbohydrates: 20g; Protein: 4g

Orange Banana Smoothie

Servings: 2
Cooking Time: 10 Minutes
Ingredients:
- 4 oranges, peeled and seeded
- 4 bananas
- 1 2-inch piece ginger root

- 2 carrots
- 2 cups of water

Directions:
1. Add all the listed ingredients to a blender
2. Blend until you have a smooth and creamy texture
3. Serve chilled and enjoy!

Nutrition Info: Calories: 164; Fat: 0.4g; Carbohydrates: 28g; Protein: 7.6g

Mango-berry Smoothie

Servings: 3
Cooking Time: 5 Minutes

Ingredients:
- ½ cup low fat plain buttermilk
- 1 cup low pat plain yogurt
- ½ lb whole strawberries
- 1 cup mango, peeled and chopped
- 1 small banana, chopped (frozen)
- 1 teaspoon raw organic honey (optional)
- 3-4 ice cubes

Directions:
1. Add everything to your blender and pulse it on high for 20 seconds and your smoothie is ready. Enjoy!

Nutrition Info: (Per Serving): Calories- 180, Fat- 15 g, Protein-5.5 g, Carbohydrates- 36.5 g

Ginger Cantaloupe Detox Smoothie

Servings: 2
Cooking Time: 10 Minutes

Ingredients:
- 1 cantaloupe, sliced
- ½ inch ginger, peeled
- 1 tablespoon flaxseed
- 1 pear, chopped
- 1 cup of water
- 1 cup ice

Directions:
1. Add all the listed ingredients to a blender except the ginger
2. Blend until smooth
3. Then add ginger and blend again
4. Serve chilled and enjoy!

Nutrition Info: Calories: 85; Fat: 2g; Carbohydrates: 19g; Protein: 2g

Berry Nectarine Smoothie

Servings: 2-3

Cooking Time: 2 Minutes

Ingredients:

- 2 nectarines, pitted and chopped
- ½ cup whole blueberries (fresh or frozen)
- ½ cup low fat plain yogurt
- ½ teaspoon vanilla extract
- 1 small banana, chopped (fresh or frozen)
- 2-3 ice cubes

Directions:

1. To you blender, add the above ingredient and pulse until smooth.

Nutrition Info: (Per Serving): Calories- 171, Fat-10 g, Protein- 4.4 g, Carbohydrates- 36 g

Berry-chard Smoothie

Servings: 3

Cooking Time: 2 Minutes

Ingredients:

- 2 cups rainbow chard, chopped
- 1 large pomegranate, peeled and seeded
- 1 cup mixed berries (fresh or frozen)
- 1 cup fresh, coconut milk
- 3-4 ice cubes

Directions:

1. Whizz all the ingredients until well combined and serve.

Nutrition Info: (Per Serving): Calories- 80, Fat- 1.5 g, Protein- 2.5 g, Carbohydrates- 41 g

The Mocha Built

Servings: 2

Cooking Time: 5 Minutes

Ingredients:

- 1 tablespoon cacao powder
- ½ cup leftover coffee
- ½ cup skim milk
- ¾ cup plain low-fat Greek yogurt
- 1 cup baby spinach
- 1 cup frozen cherries
- 1 fresh banana

Directions:

1. Add all the ingredients except vegetables/fruits first
2. Blend until smooth
3. Add the vegetable/fruits
4. Blend until smooth
5. Add a few ice cubes and serve the smoothie
6. Enjoy!

Nutrition Info: Calories: 178; Fat: 3g; Carbohydrates: 34g; Protein: 10g

Chai Coconut Shake

Servings: 1
Cooking Time: 10 Minutes
Ingredients:
- ¼ cup shredded coconut, unsweetened
- 1 cup coconut milk, unsweetened
- 1 tablespoon pure vanilla extract
- 2 tablespoons almond butter
- 1 teaspoon ginger, grounded
- 1 teaspoon cinnamon, grounded
- 1 tablespoon flaxseed, grounded
- 5 ice cubes
- Pinch of allspice

Directions:
1. Add listed ingredients to a blender
2. Blend until you have a smooth and creamy texture
3. Serve chilled and enjoy!

Nutrition Info: Calories: 233; Fat: 20g; Carbohydrates: 5g; Protein: 4g

The Pinky Swear

Servings: 2
Cooking Time: 5 Minutes
Ingredients:
- 1 pack (3.5 ounces) frozen dragon fruit
- ¾ cup low-fat Greek yogurt
- 1 cup frozen pineapple
- 1 cup unsweetened coconut milk

Directions:
1. Add all the ingredients except vegetables/fruits first
2. Blend until smooth
3. Add the vegetable/fruits
4. Blend until smooth
5. Add a few ice cubes and serve the smoothie
6. Enjoy!

Nutrition Info: Calories: 200; Fat: 3g; Carbohydrates: 36g; Protein: 6g

Ginger-mango Berry Blush

Servings: 2
Cooking Time: 2 Minutes
Ingredients:

- 1 large handful of whole strawberries (fresh or frozen)
- ½ cup mango, peeled and chopped (fresh or frozen)
- ¼ cup low fat plain yogurt
- ¼ cup filtered water
- 2-3 drops of vanilla extract
- ½ teaspoon freshly grated ginger
- 1 teaspoon raw organic honey (optional)
- 1 teaspoon freshly squeezed lemon juice
- 3-4 ice cubes

Directions:

1. Whizz all the ingredients until well combined and serve.

Nutrition Info: (Per Serving): Calories- 135, Fat- 1.1 g, Protein- 4 g, Carbohydrates- 35 g

ANTI-AGEING SMOOTHIES

Beets And Berry Beauty Enhancer

Servings: 2
Cooking Time: 5 Minutes
Ingredients:
- 1 teaspoon ginger, grated
- 2 tablespoons pumpkin seeds
- ¼ cup avocado, chopped
- ¼ cup beet, steamed and peeled
- 1/3 cup frozen strawberries
- 1/3 cup frozen raspberries
- 1/3 cup frozen blueberries
- ½ cup Greek yogurt
- ½ cup unsweetened almond milk

Directions:
1. Add all the ingredients except vegetables/fruits first
2. Blend until smooth
3. Add the vegetable/fruits
4. Blend until smooth
5. Add a few ice cubes and serve the smoothie
6. Enjoy!

Nutrition Info: Calories: 418; Fat: 20g; Carbohydrates: 50g; Protein: 17g

Green Tea-cacao Berry Smoothie

Servings: 2
Cooking Time: 10 Minutes
Ingredients:
- 1 cup unsweetened almond or soy milk
- ½ cup strawberries (fresh or frozen)
- ½ cup blueberries (fresh or frozen)
- ½ cup raspberries (fresh or frozen)
- 1/3 cup freshly brewed green tea
- 1 tablespoon cacao powder
- 3-4 ice cubes

Directions:
1. To make the green tea, first takes a sauce pan, bring the water to a boil and take it off the heat.
2. Next add the green tea bag and allow it to steep it for 5 minutes.
3. Allow the tea to cool down to room temperature.
4. Then discard the tea bag.
5. Pour all the ingredients including the tea into the blender jar and run it on medium high for 30 seconds or until smooth.

Nutrition Info: (Per Serving): Calories-121, Fat- 2.4 g, Protein- 3.6 g, Carbohydrates- 21 g

The Super Green

Servings: 1
Cooking Time: 10 Minutes
Ingredients:
- 1 tablespoon agave nectar
- 1 bunch kale, spinach, Swiss chard or combination
- 1 bunch cilantro
- 2 cucumbers, chopped and peeled
- 1 lime, peeled
- 1 lemon, outer yellow peeled
- 1 orange, peeled
- ½ cup ice

Directions:
1. Add all the listed ingredients to a blender
2. Blend until you have a smooth and creamy texture
3. Serve chilled and enjoy!

Nutrition Info: Calories: 3180; Fat: 15g; Carbohydrates: 8g; Protein: 5g

Hazelnut And Banana Crunch

Servings: 1 Large
Cooking Time: 2 Minutes
Ingredients:
- ¾ cup unsweetened almond milk
- 1 large banana, sliced (fresh or frozen)
- ¼ cup hazelnuts, chopped
- ¼ teaspoon nutmeg powder
- 1 teaspoon raw, organic honey
- 1-2 ice cubes

Directions:
1. Add everything to the blender and pulse until smooth. Serve chilled!

Nutrition Info: (Per Serving): Calories- 221, Fat- 9.5 g, Protein- 7.8 g, Carbohydrates- 25 g

The Anti-aging Avocado

Servings: 2
Cooking Time: 5 Minutes
Ingredients:
- 1 cup ice
- 1 teaspoon vanilla extract
- 1 teaspoon grapeseed oil
- ½ cup avocado, chopped
- ½ cup of frozen strawberries
- ½ cup frozen peaches, chopped
- ½ cup plain Greek yogurt
- ¼ cup 100% pomegranate juice

Directions:
1. Add all the ingredients except vegetables/fruits first
2. Blend until smooth
3. Add the vegetable/fruits
4. Blend until smooth
5. Add a few ice cubes and serve the smoothie
6. Enjoy!

Nutrition Info: Calories: 447; Fat: 23g; Carbohydrates: 39g; Protein: 22g

Carrot-beet-berry Blush

Servings: 4
Cooking Time: 5 Minutes
Ingredients:
- 2 cups fresh coconut water
- ½ cup whole raspberries (fresh or frozen)
- ½ cup whole strawberries (fresh or frozen)
- ½ cup cherries, pitted (fresh or frozen)
- ½ cup blackberries (fresh or frozen)
- 1/3 cup Goji berries
- 1 large beet, peeled and chopped
- 1 large carrot, peeled and chopped
- 1 tablespoon freshly squeezed lemon juice
- 1 tablespoon raw organic honey
- 4-5 ice cubes

Directions:
1. Combine all the ingredients in the blender and process until thick and smooth.

Nutrition Info: (Per Serving): Calories- 225, Fat- 1.7 g, Protein- 6 g, Carbohydrates-52 g

The Wrinkle Fighter

Servings: 1
Cooking Time: 10 Minutes
Ingredients:
- 2 brazil nuts
- 1 tablespoon flaxseeds
- 1 orange, peeled and cut in half
- 2 cups wild blueberries, frozen
- 2 cups kale, roughly chopped
- 1 ½ cups cold coconut water

Directions:
1. Add all the listed ingredients to a blender
2. Blend until you have a smooth and creamy texture
3. Serve chilled and enjoy!

Nutrition Info: Calories: 180; Fat: 15g; Carbohydrates: 8g; Protein: 5g

Pineapple Basil Blast

Servings: 2
Cooking Time: 5 Minutes
Ingredients:
- 1 cup pineapple, peeled and chopped
- 1 cup fresh coconut water
- Freshly squeezed juice of 1 lime
- A handful if mixed greens of your choice
- A handful of sweet basil leaves
- ¼ cup baby spinach
- 1 cup cucumber, chopped
- 1 teaspoon raw organic honey
- 1 tablespoon freshly squeezed lemon juice
- 4-5 ice cubes

Directions:
1. Pour all the ingredients into the blender and process on medium speed for 45 seconds or until the desired consistency is reached.

Nutrition Info: (Per Serving): Calories- 153, Fat- 2.5 g, Protein- 4 g, Carbohydrates- 32 g

Apple Cherry Pumpkin Tea

Servings: 2
Cooking Time: 5 Minutes
Ingredients:
- ¼ cup almonds
- ¼ cup canned pumpkin
- 1 red apple, cored, peel on
- 1 cup frozen cherries
- 1 cup brewed and chilled rooibos tea
- 1 tablespoon coconut flour
- 1 serving pea protein
- ¼ teaspoon cinnamon
- 1 pitted Medjool date
- 1 cup ice

Directions:
1. Add all the ingredients except vegetables/fruits first
2. Blend until smooth
3. Add the vegetable/fruits
4. Blend until smooth
5. Add a few ice cubes and serve the smoothie
6. Enjoy!

Nutrition Info: Calories: 534; Fat: 2g; Carbohydrates: 78g; Protein: 33g

Acai Berry And Orange Smoothie

Servings: 2

Cooking Time: 5 Minutes
Ingredients:
- 1 cup Acai berry, fresh or frozen
- ½ cup pineapple, chopped (fresh or frozen)
- 1 cup whole strawberries(fresh or frozen)
- 1 cup freshly squeezed mango juice
- 1 banana, sliced (fresh or frozen)
- 1 teaspoon agave nectar or raw organic honey
- 3-4 ice cubes

Directions:
1. Load the blender with all the ingredients and process until the smoothie has reached your desired consistency.

Nutrition Info: (Per Serving): Calories- 201, Fat- 3 g, Protein- 3.1 g, Carbohydrates- 40 g

Lychee- Cucumber Cooler

Servings: 3-4
Cooking Time: 5 Minutes
Ingredients:
- 1 ½ cup fresh coconut water
- 1 ½ cup red grapes
- 4-5 lychees, peeled and pitted
- 1 large cucumber, chopped
- 1 handful of spinach
- ½ cup of broccoli florets
- ½ cup chard or kale
- 1 tablespoon lemon juice
- 5-6 cubes of ice

Directions:
1. Place all the ingredients into your blender and run in high for 30 seconds or until smooth and frothy. Pour into glasses and serve immediately.

Nutrition Info: (Per Serving): Calories 272, - Fat- 1.6 g, Protein- 7 g, Carbohydrates- 70 g

Raspberry Goji Berry Duet

Servings: 3-4
Cooking Time: 5 Minutes
Ingredients:
- 2 cups fresh coconut water
- 1/3 cup Goji berries
- 1 cup raspberries (fresh or frozen)
- 1 avocado, peeled, pitted and chopped
- 1 large banana, sliced (fresh or frozen)
- 1 tablespoon Chia sees, soaked
- 1 tablespoon flaxseed
- 1 tablespoon raw organic honey
- 1 teaspoon freshly squeezed lemon juice

- 3-4 ice cubes

Directions:

1. Load the blender with all the ingredients listed above and pulse it on medium for 45 seconds or until done.

Nutrition Info: (Per Serving): Calories- 412, Fat- 15 g, Protein- 10 g, Carbohydrates- 65 g

The Glass Of Glowing Skin

Servings: 1
Cooking Time: 10 Minutes

Ingredients:

- ½ avocado, sliced
- 2 cups kale
- 1 cup mango, chopped
- 1 cup pineapple, chopped
- 2 frozen bananas, peeled and sliced
- ½ cup of coconut water
- 1 tablespoon flax

Directions:

1. Add all the listed ingredients to a blender
2. Blend until you have a smooth and creamy texture
3. Serve chilled and enjoy!

Nutrition Info: Calories: 430; Fat: 40g; Carbohydrates: 20g; Protein: 10g

Passion Fruit Smoothie

Servings: 4
Cooking Time: 5 Minutes

Ingredients:

- 2 ½ cups mango, chopped
- 4 passion fruits, peeled and chopped
- 1 cup unsweetened almond milk
- 1 cup plain yogurt
- Freshly squeezed juice of 1 lime
- 2 teaspoons f raw organic honey (optional)
- 5-6 ice cubes

Directions:

1. Place all the ingredients into a high speed blender and blend until everything is well combined. Serve immediately.

Nutrition Info: (Per Serving): Calories-121, Fat- 1 g, Protein- 5.7 g, Carbohydrates- 24 g

DIGESTION SUPPORT SMOOTHIES

Hemp-melon Refresher

Servings: 1-2
Cooking Time: 2 Minutes
Ingredients:
- 1 ½ cup melon, chopped
- 1 large banana, chopped
- 1 teaspoon freshly grated ginger
- 2 teaspoons hemp seed powder
- ¾ cup filtered water
- 2-4 cubes of ice
- 1 inch of cinnamon powder

Directions:
1. Place all the items listed above into the blender jar and process until the smoothie is thick and creamy.

Nutrition Info: (Per Serving): Calories- 120, Fat- 2 g, Protein- 3.1 g, Carbohydrates- 27 g

Great Green Garden

Servings: 2
Cooking Time: 5 Minutes
Ingredients:
- 1 teaspoon spirulina
- Few fresh mint leaves
- ½ cup cucumber, peeled
- ¾ cup plain coconut yogurt
- 1 cup pineapple, frozen
- 1 cup mango, frozen
- 1 cup unsweetened coconut milk

Directions:
1. Add all the ingredients except vegetables/fruits first
2. Blend until smooth
3. Add the vegetable/fruits
4. Blend until smooth
5. Add a few ice cubes and serve the smoothie
6. Enjoy!

Nutrition Info: Calories: 200; Fat: 6g; Carbohydrates: 32g; Protein: 10g

Almond And Date Smoothie

Servings: 2
Cooking Time: 5 Minutes
Ingredients:
- 1 cup unsweetened almond milk
- 3 teaspoons almond butter
- 2 cups baby spinach, washed and chopped

- 1 large apple, cored and chopped
- 1/3 teaspoon vanilla extract
- 2-3 medjool dates, pitted
- A pinch of cinnamon powder
- A pinch of Celtic salt
- 2-3 ice cubes

Directions:

1. Combine all the above listed items in the blender jar and whip it up nice and smooth. Pour into 2 servings lasses and enjoy.

Nutrition Info: (Per Serving): Calories- 500, Fat- 19 g, Protein- 11 g, Carbohydrates- 82 g

Blueberry, Oats And Chia Smoothie

Servings: 2
Cooking Time: 5 Minutes

Ingredients:

- ½ cup blueberries
- 2 tablespoons chia seeds
- ¼ cup oats
- 2 cups low-fat milk

Directions:

1. Add all the listed ingredients to a blender
2. Blend until you have a smooth and creamy texture
3. Serve chilled and enjoy!

Nutrition Info: Calories: 140; Fat: 3g; Carbohydrates: 25g; Protein: 6g

Hearty Papaya Drink

Servings: 2
Cooking Time: 5 Minutes

Ingredients:

- 1 tablespoon chia seeds
- ¾ cup plain coconut yogurt
- 1 cup baby spinach
- 1 cup frozen papaya
- 1 cup frozen tropical fruit mix
- 1 cup coconut milk, unsweetened

Directions:

1. Add all the ingredients except vegetables/fruits first
2. Blend until smooth
3. Add the vegetable/fruits
4. Blend until smooth
5. Add a few ice cubes and serve the smoothie
6. Enjoy!

Nutrition Info: Calories: 192; Fat: 7g; Carbohydrates: 31g; Protein: 3g

Spin-apple Pear Smoothie

Servings: 2-3
Cooking Time: 5 Minutes
Ingredients:
- 1 large banana, chipped
- 1 large apple, cored and chopped
- 1 pear, cored and chopped
- 2 cups baby spinach, washed and chopped
- 1 teaspoon raw organic honey (optional)
- 1 cup filtered water
- 2-4 cubes of ice
- A pinch of Celtic salt

Directions:
1. Combine everything in the blender jar and pulse until smooth and frothy.

Nutrition Info: (Per Serving): Calories- 73, Fat- 3 g, Protein- 4.2 g, Carbohydrates- 19.5 g

Noteworthy Vitamin C

Servings: 2
Cooking Time: 5 Minutes
Ingredients:
- 1 tablespoon chia seeds
- 1 clementine
- ¾ cup plain low-fat Greek yogurt
- 1 cup frozen strawberries
- 1 cup cantaloupe
- 1 cup unsweetened vanilla almond milk

Directions:
1. Add all the ingredients except vegetables/fruits first
2. Blend until smooth
3. Add the vegetable/fruits
4. Blend until smooth
5. Add a few ice cubes and serve the smoothie
6. Enjoy!

Nutrition Info: Calories: 209; Fat: 2g; Carbohydrates: 41g; Protein: 12g

Chia-berry Belly Blaster

Servings: 2
Cooking Time: 5 Minutes
Ingredients:
- 1 cup berries, frozen
- 1 cup plain Greek yogurt, unsweetened
- 1 tablespoon chia seeds, ground
- 1 tablespoon vanilla extract
- ½ cup ice

Directions:
1. Add all the listed ingredients to a blender
2. Blend until you have a smooth and creamy texture
3. Serve chilled and enjoy!

Nutrition Info: Calories: 148; Fat: 5g; Carbohydrates: 26g; Protein: 4g

Banana Oatmeal Detox Smoothie

Servings: 2
Cooking Time: 10 Minutes
Ingredients:
- 3 tablespoons collard greens
- 3 tablespoons oats
- 1 banana, peeled
- 1 apple, chopped
- 1 teaspoon cinnamon
- 1 cup ice
- 1 cup of water

Directions:
1. Add all the listed ingredients to a blender
2. Blend until you have a smooth and creamy texture
3. Serve chilled and enjoy!

Nutrition Info: Calories: 162; Fat: 1g; Carbohydrates: 41g; Protein: 3g

A Minty Drink

Servings: 2
Cooking Time: 5 Minutes
Ingredients:
- 1 tablespoon hemp seeds
- Fresh mint leaves
- ¾ cup plain coconut yogurt
- 1 cup frozen mango
- 1 cup frozen strawberries
- 1 cup unsweetened vanilla almond milk

Directions:
1. Add all the ingredients except vegetables/fruits first
2. Blend until smooth
3. Add the vegetable/fruits
4. Blend until smooth
5. Add a few ice cubes and serve the smoothie
6. Enjoy!

Nutrition Info: Calories: 391; Fat: 10g; Carbohydrates: 44g; Protein: 5g

Mango-almond Smoothie

Servings: 3-4

Cooking Time: 5 Minutes
Ingredients:
- 2 large bananas, chopped
- 2 cups mango, chopped (fresh or frozen)
- 1 cup of unsweetened almond milk
- 1 cup coconut water
- 1 teaspoon raw organic honey
- 2 teaspoon of maca root powder
- 1 teaspoon flax seed powder
- 2-3 drops of vanilla extract
- 2-3 cubes of ice

Directions:
1. Load all the ingredients into the blender and whizz it for 30 seconds until smoothie is ready.

Nutrition Info: (Per Serving): Calories- 375, Fat- 8 g, Protein- 20 g, Carbohydrates- 75 g

Coconut Berry Smoothie

Servings: 1 Large
Cooking Time: 5 Minutes
Ingredients:
- ½ cup coconut milk
- ½ cup coconut water
- 1 cup whole strawberries (fresh or frozen)
- 1 large banana, chopped
- 3 teaspoons hemp seed powder
- 1 teaspoon flax seed powder
- 1 teaspoon raw, organic honey

Directions:
1. Whizz up all the ingredients in your high speed blender for 30 seconds and serve immediately.

Nutrition Info: (Per Serving): Calories- 355, Fat- 11.5 g, Protein- 23 g, Carbohydrates- 47 g

Blueberry Chia Smoothie

Servings: 2
Cooking Time: 10 Minutes
Ingredients:
- 2 cups blueberries, frozen
- 1 cup coconut cream
- 4 tablespoons coconut oil
- 4 tablespoons swerve sweetener
- 4 tablespoons chia seeds, ground
- 2 cups full-fat Greek yogurt
- 2 cups almond milk, unsweetened

Directions:
1. Add all the listed ingredients to a blender
2. Blend until you have a smooth and creamy texture

3. Serve chilled and enjoy!
Nutrition Info: Calories: 351; Fat: 36g; Carbohydrates: 12.8g; Protein: 12.9g

Raspberry Flaxseed Smoothie

Servings: 1 Large
Cooking Time: 2 Minutes
Ingredients:
- ½ cup unsweetened almond milk
- ½ cup plain yogurt
- 1 cup raspberries (fresh or frozen)
- 1 large banana, chopped
- 1 tablespoon flaxseeds
- 1 teaspoon freshly squeezed lemon juice
- 2-3 ice cubes

Directions:
1. Place all the ingredients into the blender and puree it on high for 3 seconds until smooth and thick.
Nutrition Info: (Per Serving): Calories- 160, Fat- 2.2 g, Protein- 7.4 g, Carbohydrates- 30 g

ANTI-INFLAMMATORY SMOOTHIES

Apple, Strawberry & Beet Smoothie

Servings: 4
Cooking Time: 10 Minutes
Ingredients:
- 2 cups frozen strawberries, hulled and sliced
- 1 beet, peeled and chopped
- 1 cup apple, peeled, cored and sliced
- 3 Medjool dates, pitted and chopped
- ¼ cup extra virgin coconut oil
- ½ cup unsweetened almond milk

Directions:
1. In a high speed blender, add all ingredients and pulse till smooth.
2. Transfer into a glass and serve immediately.

Nutrition Info: (Per Serving):Calories: 223.4, Fat: 14.6g, Carbohydrates: 22.3g, Fiber: 3.9g, Protein: 1.5g, Sodium: 49.7mg

Ginger Carrot Smoothie

Servings: 2
Cooking Time: 5 Minutes
Ingredients:
- ½ cup of freshly squeezed homemade carrot juice
- 1 ripe banana, chopped
- 1 cup of pineapple, chopped
- ½ teaspoon of fresh ginger, peeled and grated
- 8 ounces of fresh almond milk (unsweetened)
- 1 ½ teaspoon of freshly squeezed lemon juice
- A pinch of turmeric powder

Directions:
1. To the blender, add all the above ingredients and run it on high for 2 minutes until all the ingredients are well combined to a creamy thick mixture.

Nutrition Info: (Per Serving): Calories-144, Fat- 2.3 g, Protein- 2.4 g Carbohydrates-32 g

Nutty Banana & Ginger Smoothie

Servings: 4
Cooking Time: 10 Minutes
Ingredients:
- 1 frozen banana, peeled and sliced
- ¼-inch fresh turmeric root, grates
- ½-inch fresh ginger root, peeled and chopped
- 1 cup pecans, chopped
- 1 cup walnuts, chopped
- 1 tablespoon flax seeds
- 1 tablespoon chia seeds

- 1 tablespoon fresh maca powder
- ½ teaspoon ground cinnamon
- 1½ cups unsweetened almond milk

Directions:
1. In a high speed blender, add all ingredients and pulse till smooth.
2. Transfer into 4 glasses and serve immediately.

Pineapple, Mango & Coconut Smoothie

Servings: 2
Cooking Time: 10 Minutes
Ingredients:
- 1 cup pineapple, chopped
- ½ cup mango, peeled, pitted and chopped
- Flesh and water of a coconut
- 1 tablespoon Goji berries
- ½ teaspoon fresh turmeric, chopped
- 1 teaspoon chia seeds
- 1 cup brewed green tea

Directions:
1. In a high speed blender, add all ingredients and pulse till smooth.
2. Transfer into 2 glasses and serve immediately.

Cherry & Blueberry Smoothie

Servings: 1
Cooking Time: 10 Minutes
Ingredients:
- 2 cups escarole
- ½ cup frozen blueberries
- ½ cup frozen cherries
- ¼ teaspoon ground cinnamon
- ¼ teaspoon ground turmeric
- 1 scoop of chocolate protein powder
- 1 cup filtered water
- 5 ice cubes, crushed

Directions:
1. In a high speed blender, add all ingredients and pulse till smooth.
2. Transfer into a glass and serve immediately.

Pina-ban-illa Smoothie

Servings: 1
Cooking Time: 5 Minutes
Ingredients:
- 1 cup pineapple, peeled and chopped

- 1 frozen banana
- 2 cups mixed green (lettuce, kale, spinach, chard etc.)
- 1 celery stalk, chopped
- 1 few drops of pure vanilla extract (or ½ organic vanilla bean)
- ¾ cup filtered water

Directions:
1. Place all the ingredients into the blender and whip it up until thick and frothy.

Nutrition Info: (Per Serving): Calories- 210, Fat- 0.7 g, Protein- 4.6 g, Carbohydrates- 55 g

Ginger-carrot Punch

Servings: 1
Cooking Time: 5 Minutes
Ingredients:
- 1 carrot, peeled and chopped
- 1 small cup of pineapple, peeled and chopped
- A handful of spinach, washed
- ½ orange, peeled and deseeded
- 1 tablespoon Chia seeds (soaked)
- ¼ teaspoon freshly grated ginger
- ½ cup of filtered water

Directions:
1. Add the washed and chopped fresh produce into the blender jar.
2. Next add the Chia seeds and water and whip up the smoothie until there are no lumps.
3. Serve.

Nutrition Info: (Per Serving): Calories-337, Fat-0 g, Protein- 8 g, Carbohydrates-52 g

3 Spice Mango Smoothie

Servings: 1
Cooking Time: 5 Minutes
Ingredients:
- ½ cup chopped mango (fresh or frozen)
- 1 bananas, chopped (fresh or frozen)
- 1 cup unsweetened almond milk
- ½ teaspoon freshly grated ginger
- ½ teaspoon freshly grated turmeric
- ½ teaspoon cinnamon powder
- ½ tablespoon of Maca root powder
- 1 tablespoon coconut oil
- ½ teaspoon of raw, organic honey
- A pinch of sea salt

Directions:
1. Place all the ingredients into your blender and run it on medium high speed for 1-2 minutes or until done.

Nutrition Info: (Per Serving): Calories-303, Fat-14g, Protein-2.8 g, Carbohydrates- 36 g

Strawberry & Kale Smoothie

Servings: 1
Cooking Time: 10 Minutes
Ingredients:
- ½ fresh strawberries, hulled and sliced
- 1 cup fresh kale, trimmed and chopped
- 1 celery stalk, chopped
- ½ of lime, peeled
- 1 cup coconut water

Directions:
1. In a high speed blender, add all ingredients and pulse till smooth.
2. Transfer into a glass and serve immediately.

Cucumber Celey Blast

Servings: 2
Cooking Time: 5 Minutes
Ingredients:
- 1 stalk celery, chopped
- ½ cup pineapple, cubed
- 1 cup green cucumber, cubed
- ¼ cup of freshly squeezed lime juice
- 1 ½ cup of coconut water
- 1 tablespoon of organic super food powder (wheatgrass, Camu root, spirulina, etc)
- 1-2 ice cubes (optional)

Directions:
1. Add all the ingredients into your blender and blend it until the desired consistency is reached.

Nutrition Info: (Per Serving): Calories- 145.2, Fats-1.7 g, Protein-4.2 g, Carbohydrates-31.6 g

Berry-beet Smoothie

Servings: 2
Cooking Time: 5 Minutes
Ingredients:
- ½ cup peeled and chopped red beet
- ½ cup chopped apple
- 1 cups strawberries (fresh or frozen)
- ¼ cup of unsweetened almond milk
- 1 tablespoon coconut oil
- 1-2 Medjool dates, pitted
- A pinch of turmeric

Directions:
1. Place all the ingredients in the blender and process it for 3-4 minutes until smooth.

Nutrition Info: (Per Serving): Calories- 223.4, Fats- 14.6 g, Protein- 1.5 g, Carbohydrates- 22.3 g

Tangy Ginger & Radish Smoothie

Servings: 2
Cooking Time: 10 Minutes
Ingredients:
- 1 orange, peeled, seeded and sliced
- 1 radish, trimmed and chopped
- 1 tablespoon fresh ginger, peeled and chopped
- 5-10 fresh mint leaves
- 1 tablespoon ground chia seeds
- 1 teaspoon organic honey
- 1 cup spring water
- ½ cup fresh orange juice
- 1 tablespoon fresh lemon juice
- Ice, as required

Directions:
1. In a high speed blender, add all ingredients and pulse till smooth.
2. Transfer into 2 glasses and serve immediately.

Sweet And Spicy Fruit Punch

Servings: 1
Cooking Time: 10 Minutes
Ingredients:
- 1 cup freshly brewed green tea (room temperature or chilled)
- ½ cup papaya, chopped (fresh or frozen)
- ½ cup avocado, chopped
- ½ cup of blueberries (fresh or frozen)
- 1 tablespoon of Chia seeds
- A handful of baby spinach
- A pinch of cayenne pepper
- ½ teaspoon of freshly grated turmeric
- ½ teaspoon of freshly grated ginger
- ½ teaspoon of cinnamon powder
- 1 teaspoon of raw, organic honey
- 1 teaspoon of coconut oil
- A pinch of sea salt

Directions:
1. Brew a fresh cup of green tea and allow it to cool.
2. If you prefer chilled smoothie, refrigerate this tea for 1 hour.
3. Next, add all the dry ingredients into the blender and process until well combined.
4. Then, pour in the wet ingredients and blend it for 30 seconds more till the desired consistency is got.
5. Serve immediately.

Nutrition Info: (Per Serving): Calories 264, Fat 13 g, Protein- 4.1 g, Carbohydrates- 41 g

Servings: 1
Cooking Time: 10 Minutes
Ingredients:
- 1-inch fresh ginger piece, peeled and chopped
- 1 frozen banana, peeled and sliced
- ½ teaspoon ground cinnamon
- 1 cup coconut milk

Directions:
1. In a high speed blender, add all ingredients and pulse till smooth.
2. Transfer into a glass and serve immediately.

MUSCLE, BONE AND JOINT SMOOTHIES

Orange Gold Smoothie

Servings: 2
Cooking Time: 5 Minutes
Ingredients:
- ½ cup fresh coconut milk
- ½ cup mango, chopped
- ½ cup pineapple, chopped
- ½ cup peaches, pitted
- ½ teaspoon freshly grated lemon zest
- ¼ teaspoon cinnamon powder
- ¼ teaspoon nutmeg powder
- ½ teaspoon cayenne pepper
- A pinch of Celtic salt
- ¾ cup filtered water
- A handful of ice cubes

Directions:
1. Place all the ingredients into the blender and whizz until thick and smooth.

Nutrition Info: (Per Serving): Calories- 171, Fat- 4.4 g, Protein- 2.9 g, Carbohydrates- 35 g

Berry-cantaloupe Smoothie

Servings: 3
Cooking Time: 5 Minutes
Ingredients:
- ½ cup whole strawberries (fresh or frozen)
- 1 cup mango, chopped
- 1 cups cantaloupe, chopped
- ½ cup fresh kale, stems removed
- 1 celery stalks, chopped
- 1 chard leaves, chopped
- A small handful of parsley
- ¼ cup baby spinach
- ½ cup filtered water

Directions:
1. Pour all the ingredients into a high speed blender and run in on high for 2 seconds or until the desired consistency is got.

Nutrition Info: (Per Serving): Calories- 375, Fat- 1.9 g, Protein- 6.8 g, Carbohydrates- 95 g

Coconut-blueberry Smoothie

Servings: 3
Cooking Time: 5 Minutes
Ingredients:
- 1 cup fresh coconut water
- 1 cup blueberries

- 1 large banana, sliced (fresh or frozen)
- 1 cup baby spinach, washed and chopped
- ½ cup fresh kale, stems removed and chopped
- ½ cup dandelion greens chopped
- 1 teaspoon freshly squeezed lemon juice

Directions:
1. Place all the ingredients into the blender and blitz until smooth.

Nutrition Info: (Per Serving): Calories- 250, Fat- 1.1 g, Protein- 4 g, Carbohydrates- 60 g

Orange Sunrise Smoothie

Servings: 3
Cooking Time: 5 Minutes
Ingredients:
- ¾ cup coconut water
- 2 large carrots, peeled and chopped
- 2 cups pineapple, chopped
- 1 cup freshly squeezed orange juice
- 1 cup lightly packed iceberg lettuce
- 2-3 celery stalks chopped
- 3 teaspoons Chia seeds, soaked
- ½ teaspoon freshly grated ginger

Directions:
1. To the blender, add all the ingredients and pulse until smooth.

Nutrition Info: (Per Serving): Calories- 345, Fat- 3 g, Protein- 7.5 g, Carbohydrates- 55g

Ginger- Parsely Grape Smoothie

Servings: 1
Cooking Time: 2 Minutes
Ingredients:
- 1 ½ cup red grapes, seedless
- ½ cup parsley, washed and chopped
- 2 tablespoons avocado flesh
- ¼ cup freshly squeezed lemon juice
- 1 teaspoon freshly grated ginger
- 3 drops of liquid Stevia or ½ teaspoon raw organic honey
- 4-5 mint leaves
- A handful of ice cubes

Directions:
1. Add all the ingredients into the blender and blitz until smooth.

Nutrition Info: (Per Serving): Calories- 230, Fat- 5.4 g, Protein- 3.9 g, Carbohydrates- 55 g

Cucumber- Pineapple

Servings: 3

Cooking Time: 5 Minutes
Ingredients:
- 1 ¼ cups fresh coconut water
- 1 cup cucumber, chopped
- ½ cup pineapple, chopped
- 1 small avocado, peeled and chopped
- 1/3 cup fresh kale, stems removed
- 1/3 cup baby spinach
- ½ teaspoon freshly grated ginger

Directions:
1. Combine all the ingredients in a high speed blender and pulse until smooth.

Nutrition Info: (Per Serving): Calories- 260, Fat- 15 g, Protein- 7 g, Carbohydrates- 22 g

Orange Kiwi Punch

Servings: 2-3
Cooking Time: 5 Minutes
Ingredients:
- 1 cup freshly squeezed orange juice
- 1 cup mango, copped
- 2 kiwi fruits, peeled and chopped
- ½ cup arugula
- ½ cup ice berg lettuce
- 1 cup fresh kale, stems removed and chopped
- 1 teaspoon flax seed powder
- 3-4 ice cubes

Directions:
1. Place all the ingredients in the blender and process until your desired consistency has reached.

Nutrition Info: (Per Serving): Calories- 350, Fat- 2 g, Protein- 7g, Carbohydrates- 85 g

Cucumber- Pear Healer

Servings: 2
Cooking Time: 2 Minutes
Ingredients:
- 1 cup unsweetened almond milk
- 2 cups cucumber, chopped
- 2 large pears, cored and chopped
- 8-9 fresh mint leaves
- 1 teaspoon freshly squeezed lemon juice
- 1 teaspoon raw organic honey
- 3-4 ice cubes

Directions:
1. Just add all the ingredients into the blender and pulse until smooth.

Nutrition Info: (Per Serving): Calories- 285, Fat- 4.8 g, Protein- 5 g, Carbohydrates- 65 g

Cilantro- Grapefriut Smoothie

Servings: 2-3
Cooking Time: 2 Minutes
Ingredients:
- 1 grapefruit, peeled and chopped
- ½ cup fresh cilantro, chopped
- 1 cup pineapple, peeled and chopped
- 1 small banana, chopped (fresh or frozen)
- 1 cup cucumber, chopped
- 1 tablespoon freshly squeezed lemon juice
- ¾ cup water
- 3-4 ice cubes

Directions:
1. To your high speed blender jar, add all the items mentioned above and process until the smoothie is thick and frothy. Pour into serving glasses and enjoy.
Nutrition Info: (Per Serving): Calories- 260, Fat- 0.2 g, Protein- 3.8 g, Carbohydrates- 68 g

Ginger Lime Smoothie

Servings: 3
Cooking Time: 5 Minutes
Ingredients:
- 1 cup fresh coconut water
- Freshly squeezed juice of 1 lime
- 1 cup pineapple, chopped
- 1 cup kale, stems removed and chopped
- ½ banana, chopped (fresh or frozen)
- ½ cup arugula
- 1-2 celery stalks, chopped
- 6-7 mint leaves
- ½ teaspoon freshly grated ginger
- 1 ½ teaspoon Chia seeds, soaked
- 2-4 ice cubes

Directions:
1. Place all the above listed ingredients into your blender and blend until smooth. Enjoy immediately.
Nutrition Info: (Per Serving): Calories- 345, Fat- 4 g, Protein- 8.5 g, Carbohydrates- 75 g

Kiwi Quick Smoothie

Servings: 2
Cooking Time: 2 Minutes
Ingredients:
- ½ cup unsweetened almond milk
- ½ cup plain yoghurt
- ¼ cup fresh coconut milk

- ½ cup whole strawberries (fresh or frozen)
- 1 kiwi, peeled and chopped
- 1 teaspoon raw, organic honey
- ½ teaspoon Chia seeds

Directions:
1. Combine all the ingredients in a high speed blender and process until smooth.

Nutrition Info: (Per Serving): Calories- 260, Fat- 9 g, Protein- 13 g, Carbohydrates- 37 g

Apple –kiwi Blush

Servings: 2
Cooking Time: 5 Minutes
Ingredients:
- 1 cup unsweetened almond milk
- 1 large apple, cored and chopped
- 2 kiwi fruits, peeled and chopped
- 1 cup cucumber, chopped
- 2-3 collard green leaves, stems removed and chopped
- 3 teaspoons Chia seeds, soaked
- 2-3 ice cubes (optional)

Directions:
1. Place all the ingredients in a high speed bender and blitz on medium speed for 30 seconds or until smooth.

Nutrition Info: (Per Serving): Calories- 340, Fat- 0.5 g, Protein- 11 g, Carbohydrates- 60 g

Pineapple Sage Smoothie

Servings: 2
Cooking Time: 5 Minutes
Ingredients:
- 1 cup pineapple, peeled and chopped
- 1 pear, core and chopped
- 2-3 sage leaves
- 1 teaspoon Chia seeds, soaked
- 1 teaspoon hemp seed powder
- 1 teaspoon freshly squeezed lemon juice
- ¾ cup water
- 2-3 ice cubes

Directions:
1. Add all the ingredients into the blender and run it on high for 30 seconds or until well combined.

Nutrition Info: (Per Serving): Calories- 250, Fat- 1.1 g, Protein- 5 g , Carbohydrates- 87 g

Fruit "n" Nut Smoothie

Servings: 2

Cooking Time: 5 Minutes
Ingredients:
- 1 cup freshly brewed green tea
- 1 cup red cherries, pitted
- 1 cup whole strawberries (fresh or frozen)
- ½ kale, stems removed
- ¼ cup walnuts, halved
- ½ teaspoon freshly grated ginger
- 1 teaspoon wheat grass powder
- 1 teaspoon hemp powder

Directions:
1. Load all the ingredients in a high speed blender and process until it is smooth and thick.

Nutrition Info: (Per Serving): Calories- 255, Fat- 11 g, Protein- 8.9 g, Carbohydrates- 38 g

SUPERFOOD SMOOTHIES

Carrot Crunch Smoothie

Servings: 2
Cooking Time: 5 Minutes
Ingredients:
- 1 grapefruit, peeled and seeded
- 1 cup carrot, peeled and chopped
- 1 cup low fat plain yogurt
- 2 teaspoons raw, organic honey
- 3 teaspoons macadamia nuts, chopped
- 3 teaspoons almonds, chopped
- 5-6 ice cubes

Directions:
1. Place all the ingredients into the high speed blender jar and run it on high for 20 seconds until everything is well combined. Pour into serving glass and enjoy!

Nutrition Info: (Per Serving): Calories- 310, Fat- 12 g, Protein- 11 g, Carbohydrates- 39 g

Tea And Grape Smoothie

Servings: 2
Cooking Time: 5 Minutes
Ingredients:
- 1 large apple, cored and chopped
- 1 cup red grapes, seedless
- ½ cup freshly brewed green tea (unsweetened and chilled)
- ½ cup plain low fat yogurt
- 1 teaspoons raw organic honey
- 1 teaspoons freshly grated ginger
- 3-4 ice cubes

Directions:
1. Load your high speed blender jar with all the ingredients and puree until thick and smooth.

Nutrition Info: (Per Serving): Calories- 131, Fat- 1 g, Protein- 5 g, Carbohydrates- 25 g

Aloe Vera Smoothie

Servings: 3
Cooking Time: 5 Minutes
Ingredients:
- ½ cup pure aloe Vera gel
- ½ ripe avocado, peeled and pitted
- Freshly squeezed juice of ½ lime
- 1 ½ teaspoon pure coconut oil
- 1 cup mixed greens, washed and chopped
- 1 kiwi, peeled and chopped
- 1 teaspoon flax seed powder
- 1 teaspoon Chia seeds

- A pinch of Celtic salt
- 1 teaspoon raw organic honey
- 1 cup filtered water
- 4-5 ice cubes
- 1 teaspoon freshly squeezed lemon juice

Directions:
1. Add all the ingredients in the same order as listed above and blend until smooth and thick

Nutrition Info: (Per Serving): Calories- 360, Fat- 31 g, Protein- 3.2 g, Carbohydrates- 35 g

Berry Melon Green Smoothie

Servings: 3
Cooking Time: 5 Minutes
Ingredients:
- ¾ cup watermelon, chopped
- ½ cup whole strawberries (fresh or frozen)
- 1 ½ cup fresh baby spinach, washed and chopped
- 1 ripe banana, chopped
- 1 cup fresh coconut water
- Freshly squeezed juice of ½ lime
- 1 ½ teaspoon flaxseed powder
- 3-4 ice cubes

Directions:
1. Add all the ingredients in the same order as listed above and blend until smooth and thick

Nutrition Info: (Per Serving): Calories- 121, Fat- 1.5 g, Protein- 3 g, Carbohydrates- 25 g

Coconut Blue Wonder

Servings: 2
Cooking Time: 5 Minutes
Ingredients:
- 1 cup whole blueberries (fresh or frozen)
- 1 cup organic coconut milk
- ¼ cup plain low fat yogurt
- 1 small handful of baby spinach, chopped
- 1 ½ teaspoon flaxseed powder
- 3-4 ice cubes

Directions:
1. Combine all the ingredients in a blender jar and run it for 1 minute or until smooth and creamy.

Nutrition Info: (Per Serving): Calories- 240, Fat- 11 g, Protein- 4 g, Carbohydrates- 31 g

Green Chia Smoothie

Servings: 3
Cooking Time: 5 Minutes

Ingredients:
- 1 ½ cups spinach, washed and chopped
- 1 large kale leaf, chopped
- 1 cup English cucumber, chopped
- 1 small apple, cored and chopped
- 1 teaspoon freshly squeezed lemon juice
- 3 teaspoons Chia seeds, soaked
- 1 teaspoon raw organic honey
- 1 ½ cup filtered water
- 3-4 ice cubes

Directions:
1. To you blender, add the above ingredient and pulse until smooth.

Nutrition Info: (Per Serving): Calories- 100, Fat- 2.9 g, Protein- 5 g, Carbohydrates- 18.5 g

Chia Flax Berry Green Smoothie

Servings: 3
Cooking Time: 5 Minutes

Ingredients:
- 1 cup unsweetened almond milk
- 2 teaspoons almond butter
- 1 cup frozen mixed berries
- 1 ripe banana, chopped
- 1 cup fresh spinach, chopped
- 2 teaspoons flaxseed powder
- 2 teaspoons Chia seeds oaked
- 1 teaspoon raw organic honey
- 4-5 ice cubes

Directions:
1. Whizz all the ingredients until well combined and serve.

Nutrition Info: (Per Serving): Calories- 360, Fat- 1.3 g, Protein- 11 g, Carbohydrates- 45 g

Basil- Bee Pollen Chlorella Smoothie

Servings: 2-3
Cooking Time: 5 Minutes

Ingredients:
- ½ cup pineapple, peeled and chopped
- 1 cup fresh coconut water
- 2 tablespoon ripe avocado flesh
- 1/3 cup low fat plain yogurt
- 1 teaspoon cacao powder
- 2 teaspoon coconut flakes
- 1 teaspoon raw organic honey
- 1 teaspoon bee pollen
- 1 teaspoon Chia seeds

- 1 teaspoon chlorella
- 1 teaspoon maca root powder
- 1 teaspoon freshly squeezed lemon juice
- 5-6 fresh basil leaves
- 1 teaspoon freshly squeezed lemon juice
- A pinch of Himalayan salt
- 4-5 ice cubes

Directions:

1. In a blender, combine all the above listed ingredients and blend until nice and smooth.

Nutrition Info: (Per Serving): Calories- 320, Fat- 14 g, Protein- 14 g, Carbohydrates- 40 g

Raspberry Carrot Smoothie

Servings: 2
Cooking Time: 5 Minutes

Ingredients:

- 1 large carrot, peeled and chopped
- 1 cup whole raspberries (fresh or frozen)
- ½ cup low fat plain yogurt
- 4 teaspoons Goji berries
- 1 tablespoon Chia seeds
- 1 tablespoon flaxseed powder
- 1 teaspoon raw organic honey
- 4-5 ice cubes

Directions:

1. To your high speed blender, add all the ingredients and pulse until smooth.

Nutrition Info: (Per Serving): Calories- 335, Fat- 12 g, Protein- 13.5 g, Carbohydrates- 45 g

Raspberry Peach Delight

Servings: 3
Cooking Time: 5 Minutes

Ingredients:

- 1 cup whole raspberries (fresh or frozen)
- 1 ½ cups peaches, pitted (fresh or frozen)
- 1 cup unsweetened, organic coconut milk
- ¼ teaspoon vanilla extract
- 2 teaspoons Chia seeds
- 2 teaspoons freshly squeezed lemon juice
- 2 teaspoons raw organic honey
- 1 cups filtered water
- 4-5 ice cubes

Directions:

1. To you blender, add the above ingredient and pulse until smooth.

Nutrition Info: (Per Serving): Calories- 161, Fat- 4.9 g, Protein- 3 g, Carbohydrates- 30 g

Banana-sunflower Coconut Smoothie

Servings: 2
Cooking Time: 2 Minutes
Ingredients:
- 2 ripe bananas, sliced (fresh or frozen)
- 3 teaspoons raw cacao powder
- 2 teaspoons maca powder
- 3 teaspoons coconut cream
- 2 teaspoon sunflower seeds
- 1 cup filtered water
- 1 teaspoon raw organic honey
- 4-5 ice cubes

Directions:
1. Place all the ingredients into your blender and run it on medium high speed for 1-2 minutes or until done.
Nutrition Info: (Per Serving): Calories- 200, Fat- 6.9 g, Protein- 3.6 g, Carbohydrates- 32 g

Blue And Green Wonder

Servings: 3
Cooking Time: 5 Minutes
Ingredients:
- 1 cup unsweetened almond milk
- 1 cup whole blueberries (fresh or frozen)
- 1 ripe banana, chopped
- 1 cup baby spinach, washed and chopped
- 1 cup fresh kale, stems removed and chopped
- 2 teaspoons flax seeds
- 4-5 ice cubes

Directions:
1. Add all the ingredients in the same order as listed above and blend until smooth and thick
Nutrition Info: (Per Serving): Calories- 122, Fat- 2 g, Protein- 3 g, Carbohydrates- 25 g

GREEN SMOOTHIES

Pineapple And Cucumber Cooler

Servings: 3-4
Cooking Time: 5 Minutes
Ingredients:
- 1 green apple, cored and chopped
- 1 cup pineapple, peeled and chopped
- 1 green cucumber, deseeded and chopped
- 5-6 celery stalks, chopped
- A handful of kale leaves, stems removed and chopped
- 1/3 cup fresh parsley
- 1 teaspoon freshly grated ginger
- 1 tablespoon freshly squeezed lemon juice
- 3-4 ice cubes

Directions:
1. Add all the ingredients into the blender jar and pulse it on high for 30 seconds or until smooth.

Nutrition Info: (Per Serving): Calories-226, Fat- 1.8 g, Protein- 7.8 g, Carbohydrates- 36 g

Tropical Apple Coconut Green Blend

Servings: 3
Cooking Time: 5 Minutes
Ingredients:
- 1 cup plain low fat yogurt
- ½ cup cucumber, deseeded and chopped
- Freshly squeezed juice of 1 lime
- 1 large green apple, cored and chopped
- ½ cup fresh coconut water
- A handful of spinach, washed and chopped
- 6-7 fresh mint leaves
- 6-7 ice cubes
- 1 teaspoon raw organic honey (optional)

Directions:
1. Pour the ingredients into the blender and process until smooth.

Nutrition Info: (Per Serving): Calories- 158, Fat- 0.3 g, Protein- 12 g, Carbohydrates- 30 g

Cilantro And Citrus Glass

Servings: 2
Cooking Time: 5 Minutes
Ingredients:
- ½ cup ice
- 2 cups arugula
- ½ cup celery, diced
- 1 grapefruit, peeled and segmented

- 1 handful fresh cilantro leaves, chopped
- ½ lemon, juiced
- ½ cup water

Directions:
1. Add all the ingredients except vegetables/fruits first
2. Blend until smooth
3. Add the vegetable/fruits
4. Blend until smooth
5. Add a few ice cubes and serve the smoothie
6. Enjoy!

Nutrition Info: Calories: 75; Fat: 1g; Carbohydrates: 16g; Protein: 3g

Cacao Mango Green Smoothie

Servings: 4
Cooking Time: 2 Minutes
Ingredients:
- 1 cup mango, peeled and chopped
- 1 cup unsweetened almond milk
- 1 cup blueberries (fresh or frozen)
- 2 cups fresh baby spinach
- 1 cup mixed greens
- 2 teaspoons Chia seeds, soaked
- 3 teaspoons raw cacao powder
- 1 teaspoon raw organic honey
- 1 teaspoon flaxseed powder
- 3-4 ice cubes

Directions:
1. Blend all the ingredients into the blender and enjoy!

Nutrition Info: (Per Serving): Calories- 339, Fat- 2.8 g, Protein- 10 g, Carbohydrates- 70 g

Lovely Green Gazpacho

Servings: 2
Cooking Time: 5 Minutes
Ingredients:
- ½ cup ice
- 1 cup collard greens, chopped
- ¼ cup red bell pepper, diced
- ½ cup frozen broccoli florets
- ½ cup fresh tomatoes, chopped
- 1 garlic clove
- ¼ cup fresh cilantro, chopped
- ½ lemon, juiced
- ½ cup water

Directions:
1. Add all the ingredients except vegetables/fruits first

2. Blend until smooth
3. Add the vegetable/fruits
4. Blend until smooth
5. Add a few ice cubes and serve the smoothie
6. Enjoy!
Nutrition Info: Calories: 70; Fat: 1g; Carbohydrates: 13g; Protein: 4g

Date And Apricot Green Smoothie

Servings: 2 Large
Cooking Time: 2 Minutes
Ingredients:
- ¾ cup unsweetened almond milk
- 1 small apricot, pitted and chopped
- 1 medjool dates, pitted
- 1 small banana, chopped
- ½ cup kale, stems removed and chopped
- ½ cup baby spinach, washed
- A handful of mixed berries
- Few ice cubes

Directions:
1. Pour the ingredients into the blender and process until smooth.
Nutrition Info: (Per Serving): Calories- 202, Fat- 3.6 g, Protein- 7.6 g, Carbohydrates- 38 g

Dandellion Green Berry Smoothie

Servings: 2
Cooking Time: 5 Minutes
Ingredients:
- ½ cup dandelion greens, chopped
- ½ small banana, hopped
- A handful of mixed berries
- 1 cup filtered water
- 1 teaspoon coconut oil
- A pinch of cinnamon powder
- 1 teaspoon flax seed powder
- 1 teaspoon cacao powder
- 1 teaspoon raw organic honey
- ½ teaspoon Chia seeds
- ½ teaspoon hemp seeds
- 3-4 ice cubes

Directions:
1. Add all the above listed ingredients into your blender, secure the lid and blitz until smooth.
Nutrition Info: (Per Serving): Calories- 270, Fat- 16 g, Protein- 3.2 g, Carbohydrates- 35 g

Clementine Green Smoothie

Servings: 3
Cooking Time: 5 Minutes
Ingredients:
- 2-3 Clementine, peeled and deseeded
- 1 small banana, chopped
- ¼ cup fresh coconut milk
- 1 small handful of mixed greens
- A few sprigs of mint leaves
- A few fresh cilantro leaves
- ½ teaspoon raw organic honey
- 1 teaspoon freshly squeezed lemon juice
- 3-4 ice cubes

Directions:
1. Add all the ingredients into the high speed blender and whizz until smooth.

Nutrition Info: (Per Serving): Calories- 180, Fat- 3.2 g, Protein- 3.5 g, Carbohydrates- 42 g

A Mean Green Milk Shake

Servings: 1
Cooking Time: 10 Minutes
Ingredients:
- 1 cup whole milk
- 1 tablespoon coconut flakes, unsweetened
- 1 cup of water
- 2 cups spring mix salad
- 1 tablespoon coconut oil
- 1 pack stevia

Directions:
1. Add listed ingredients to a blender
2. Blend until you have a smooth and creamy texture
3. Serve chilled and enjoy!

Nutrition Info: Calories: 309; Fat: 23g; Carbohydrates: 18g; Protein: 9.5g

The Minty Cucumber

Servings: 2
Cooking Time: 5 Minutes
Ingredients:
- ½ cup ice
- 1½ cups swiss chard, chopped
- ¾ cup cucumber, diced
- 1 pear, roughly chopped
- ¼ cup fresh cilantro, chopped
- 4 fresh mint leaves, chopped
- ½ lemon, juiced

- ¼ cup water

Directions:
1. Add all the ingredients except vegetables/fruits first
2. Blend until smooth
3. Add the vegetable/fruits
4. Blend until smooth
5. Add a few ice cubes and serve the smoothie
6. Enjoy

Nutrition Info: Calories: 105; Fat: 0g; Carbohydrates: 25g; Protein: 3g

Berry Spinach Basil Smoothie

Servings: 2
Cooking Time: 5 Minutes
Ingredients:
- 1 cup unsweetened almond milk
- 1 small banana, chopped
- ½ cup blueberries (fresh or frozen)
- A small handful of baby spinach
- 6-7 fresh basil leaves
- 2 teaspoons freshly squeezed lemon juice
- 3-4 ice cubes

Directions:
1. Add all the ingredients into the high speed blender and whizz until smooth.

Nutrition Info: (Per Serving): Calories- 250, Fat- 5.8g, Protein- 5 g ,Carbohydrates- 51 g

Coco-banann Green Smoothie

Servings: 3
Cooking Time: 5 Minutes
Ingredients:
- 1 cup fresh kale, stems removed and chopped
- 1 cup baby spinach, washed
- 1 ½ cups pineapple, peeled and chopped
- ½ cup fresh coconut milk
- 1 large ripe banana, chopped
- 2 tablespoons freshly squeezed lime juice
- 1 tablespoon fresh parsley
- 3-4 ice cubes

Directions:
1. To make this smoothie, place everything into the blender and pulse until smooth. Serve immediately.

Nutrition Info: (Per Serving): Calories-250, Fat-12.7 g, Protein- 4.7 g, Carbohydrates- 35 g

Banana Green Smoothie

Servings: 2

Cooking Time: 10 Minutes
Ingredients:
- 2 bananas
- 1 cup strawberries
- 1 cup almond milk
- 2 cups spinach, raw
- 2 teaspoons vanilla extract

Directions:
1. Add listed ingredients to a blender
2. Blend until you have a smooth and creamy texture
3. Serve chilled and enjoy!

Nutrition Info: Calories: 212; Fat: 14.7g; Carbohydrates: 20.4g; Protein: 2.7g

Glowing Green Smoothie

Servings: 2
Cooking Time: 10 Minutes
Ingredients:
- 2 bananas
- 2 kiwis
- 4 celery stalks
- ½ cup pineapple
- 2 cups of water
- 4 cups spinach

Directions:
1. Add all the listed ingredients to a blender
2. Blend until you have a smooth and creamy texture
3. Serve chilled and enjoy!

Nutrition Info: Calories: 191; Fat: 1.1g; Carbohydrates: 46.5g; Protein: 7.8g

VEGAN AND VEGETARIAN DIET SMOOTHIES

Beet And Grapefruit Smoothie

Servings: 1
Cooking Time: 5 Min
Ingredients:
- 1/2 Cucumber, peeled and diced
- 1/2 small red beet, peeled and diced
- 1 apple, cored and chopped
- 6 tbsps. Grapefruit juice
- 4 ice cubes

Directions:
1. In a high speed blender, add cucumber and blend until it breaks into pieces. Add apple, beet and blend until smooth.
2. Add water if it's too hard to blend. Push the sides and blend again until you reach fine consistency. Add ice, grapefruit juice and blend.
3. Serve right away.

Nutrition Info: (Per Serving): Cal 208 Total Fat 1.2 g, Carbs 45.9 g, Fiber 4 g, Protein 6 g, Sodium 33 mg Sugars 25 g

Pina Colada Smoothie

Servings: 2
Cooking Time: 5 Min
Ingredients:
- 1 cup pineapple chunks
- 1 banana
- 2 teaspoons honey
- 1 cup reduced fat coconut milk, unsweetened
- ½ cup ice cubes
- 2 Pineapple wedges, for garnish

Directions:
1. Peel banana, chop roughly and place in a blender along with pineapple, honey, coconut milk and ice cubes.
2. Pulse for 1 minute until smooth and divide smoothie between two serving glasses.
3. Garnish each serving glass with a pineapple wedge and serve immediately.

Nutrition Info: (Per Serving):158 Cal, 6.6 g total fat (2 g sat. fat), 0 mg chol., 39 mg sodium, 23 g carb., 2g fiber, 2.7 g protein.

Spinach, Grape, & Coconut Smoothie

Servings: 2
Cooking Time: 5 Min
Ingredients:
- 2 cups seedless green grapes
- 2 cups baby spinach
- ½ cup reduced fat coconut milk
- 1 cup ice cubes

Directions:
1. In a blender, place grapes, spinach and ice, and pour in milk.

2. Pulse for 1 minute until smooth and serve immediately.
Nutrition Info: (Per Serving):194 Cal, 2 g total fat (0 g sat. fat), 0 mg chol., 108 mg sodium, 31 g carb., 4g fiber, 0 g protein.

Apple, Carrot, Ginger & Fennel Smoothie

Servings: 2
Cooking Time: 5 Min
Ingredients:
- 1 medium apple
- 2 medium carrots
- 2 tablespoons peeled ginger slices
- 1 cup sliced fennel bulb
- 1 tablespoon honey
- 1 cup apple juice
- 1 tablespoons lemon juice
- 1 cup ice cubes

Directions:
1. Peel and core apple, cut into slices and place in a blender.
2. Peel carrots, dice and add to blender along with ginger, fennel bulb, honey, apple juice, lemon juice and ice cubes.
3. Pulse for 1 minute until smoothie and serve immediately.
Nutrition Info: (Per Serving):144 Cal, 0 g total fat (0 g sat. fat), 0 mg chol., 63 mg sodium, 36 g carb., 5g fiber, 2 g protein.

Super Avocado Smoothie

Servings: 2
Cooking Time: 5 Min
Ingredients:
- 1 medium avocado
- 1 cup blueberries
- 1 cup frozen strawberries
- ½ cup frozen raspberries
- ¼ cup reduced fat vanilla yogurt
- 1 cup orange juice
- ½ cup filtered water
- 1 tablespoon maple syrup
- 15 mint leaves

Directions:
1. Peel and pit avocado and add to a blender.
2. Add blueberries, strawberries, raspberries, yogurt, orange juice, water, maple syrup and mint.
3. Pulse for 1 minute until smooth and serve immediately.
Nutrition Info: (Per Serving):156 Cal, 8 g total fat (1 g sat. fat), 0 mg chol., 64 mg sodium, 54 g carb., 8g fiber, 3 g protein.

Chia, Blueberry & Banana Smoothie

Servings: 2

Cooking Time: 5 Min
Ingredients:
- 2 medium fresh bananas
- 1 cup frozen blueberries
- 1 cup fat free milk, unsweetened
- 2 tablespoons Chia Seeds
- 1 cup ice cubes

Directions:
1. Peel banana, chop roughly and place in a blender along with blueberries, milk, chia seeds and ice.
2. Pulse 1 minute until smooth and serve immediately.

Nutrition Info: (Per Serving):220 Cal, 1.5 g total fat (0.5 g sat. fat), 0 mg chol., 71 mg sodium, 48 g carb., 3.4g fiber, 5.5 g protein.

Green Smoothie

Servings: 2
Cooking Time: 5 Min
Ingredients:
- 2 medium green apples
- Half of a medium avocado
- 1-inch ginger piece
- 1 cup baby spinach
- 1 cup coconut water
- 1 tablespoon flax oil
- 1 cup ice cubes

Directions:
1. Peel apple, core, slice and place in a blender. Peel and pit avocado and add to blender.
2. Peel and dice ginger and add to blender along with spinach, coconut water, flax oil and ice cubes.
3. Pulse for 1 minute until smooth and creamy and then serve over ice.

Nutrition Info: (Per Serving):156 Cal, 1 g total fat (0.2 g sat. fat), 0 mg chol., 54 mg sodium, 38 g carb., 6.5g fiber, 3.6 g protein.

Strawberry Watermelon Smoothie

Servings: 2
Cooking Time: 5 Min
Ingredients:
- 1 1/2 cups sliced watermelons, seeds removed
- 1 cup frozen strawberries
- 1/2 frozen ripe banana, sliced
- 1/2 cup unsweetened almond milk
- 1 lime juice
- 1 tbsp. chia seeds

Directions:
1. Add all ingredients in a blender. Process until smooth and fine texture. Adjust sweetness with more banana.
2. Top with more chia seeds.

Nutrition Info: (Per Serving): Cal 182 Total Fat 6.2 g, Carbs 30 g, Fiber 9 g, Protein 5 g, Sodium 48 mg Sugars 14 g

Healthy Kiwi Smoothie

Servings: 2
Cooking Time: 20 Min
Ingredients:
- 1 celery stalk
- 2 medium granny smith apples, cored
- 1 kiwi fruit, peeled and chopped
- 1/3 cup parsley leaves
- 1 tbsp. grated ginger
- Maple syrup
- 2 tsp lime juice

Directions:
1. Add all ingredients in a blender, except lime juice and blend until smooth. Taste and adjust sweetness with maple syrup.
2. Stir in lime juice and serve.

Nutrition Info: (Per Serving): Cal 82 Total Fat 1 g, Carbs 20 g, Fiber 0 g, Protein 1 g, Sodium 9 mg Sugars 18 g

Lime & Green Tea Smoothie Bowl

Servings: 2
Cooking Time: 10 Min
Ingredients:
- 1/2 cup coconut juice/ water
- 1 cup fresh spinach leaves
- 1 large frozen banana slices
- 1/4 cup avocado slices
- 2 tsp lime zest
- 1 tbsp. and 1 tsp lime juice
- 3 ice cubes
- 2 tsp maple syrup
- 1/2 tsp good quality Matcha Green Tea powder
- Toppings:
- Granola, chopped into pieces
- Coconut flakes
- Coconut cream

Directions:
1. Put all the ingredients in a high-speed blender, except the toppings. Blend until smooth.
2. Transfer in glasses or bowls. Put toppings as much as you want. Enjoy!

Nutrition Info: (Per Serving): Cal 437 Total Fat 22.4 g, Carbs 55.4 g, Fiber 10.9 g, Protein 10.4 g, Sodium 44 mg Sugars 31.9 g

BRAIN HEALTH SMOOTHIES

Pear 'n' Kale Smoothie

Servings: 2-3
Cooking Time: 5 Minutes
Ingredients:
- 1 large pear, peeled, cored and chopped
- 1 green apple, peeled, cored and chopped
- ½ cup pineapple, peeled and chipped
- 1 cup fresh kale, stems removed and chopped
- 1 cup mixed greens, washed and chopped
- 1 tablespoon freshly squeezed lemon juice
- 4 ounces of filtered water

Directions:
1. Combine all the ingredients in the blender and whip it on high for 30 seconds till the smoothie is thick and well combined.
Nutrition Info: (Per Serving): Calories- 250, Fat- 1.2 g, Protein- 3.2 g, Carbohydrates- 64 g

3 Spice-almond Smoothie

Servings: 1 Large
Cooking Time: 5 Minutes
Ingredients:
- ¾ cup unsweetened almond milk
- 1 banana, sliced (fresh or frozen)
- A handful of fresh kale, stems removed
- 1 teaspoon almond butter
- A pinch of nutmeg powder
- 1 pinch of cinnamon powder
- ¼ teaspoon of freshly grated ginger
- ½ teaspoon of raw organic honey

Directions:
1. Place all the ingredients into the high speed blender jar and run it on high for 20 seconds until everything is well combined. Pour into serving glass and enjoy!
Nutrition Info: (Per Serving): Calories- 238, Fat- 10 g, Protein- 5.5 g, Carbohydrates- 39 g

Pomegranate, Tangerine And Ginger Smoothie

Servings: 2
Cooking Time: 5 Minutes
Ingredients:
- ½ cup pomegranate
- 1-inch ginger root, crushed
- 1 cup tangerine
- A pinch of Himalayan pink salt

Directions:
1. Toss the pomegranate, ginger roots and tangerine into your blender

2. Add a pinch of Himalayan salt
3. Serve chilled and enjoy!
Nutrition Info: Calories: 121; Fat: 6g; Carbohydrates: 20g; Protein: 4g

Berry Berry Smoothie

Servings: 4
Cooking Time: 10 Minutes
Ingredients:
- 2 bananas
- 3 cups blueberries, frozen
- 2 cups almond milk
- 2 tablespoons almond butter
- 2 handfuls ice

Directions:
1. Add all the listed ingredients to a blender
2. Blend until you have a smooth and creamy texture
3. Serve chilled and enjoy!
Nutrition Info: Calories: 352; Fat: 27g; Carbohydrates: 41.5g; Protein: 4.7g

Berry Infusion Smoothie

Servings: 2
Cooking Time: 2 Minutes
Ingredients:
- ½ cup freshly prepared pomegranate juice
- ½ large banana, chopped (fresh or frozen)
- ½ cup blueberries (fresh or frozen)
- ½ cup raspberries (fresh or frozen)
- A handful of pineapple chunks
- 2 tablespoons Chia seeds, soaked
- A few ice cubes

Directions:
1. Add all the ingredients into your blender jar, secure the lid firmly and whizz for 30 seconds or until the smoothie is thick and creamy.
Nutrition Info: (Per Serving): Calories- 378, Fat- 4.5 g, Protein- 25 g, Carbohydrates- 68 g

Matcha Coconut Smoothie

Servings: 2
Cooking Time: 5 Minutes
Ingredients:
- 3 tablespoons white beans
- ½ teaspoon matcha green tea powder
- 1 whole banana, cubed
- 1 cup of frozen mango, chunked

- 2 kale leaves, torn
- 2 tablespoon coconut, shredded
- 1 cup of water

Directions:
1. Add all the listed ingredients to a blender
2. Blend on high until you have a smooth and creamy texture
3. Serve chilled and enjoy!

Nutrition Info: Calories: 291; Fat: 25g; Carbohydrates: 18g; Protein: 5g

The Gritty Coffee Shake

Servings: 1
Cooking Time: 10 Minutes
Ingredients:
- 2 cups strongly brewed coffee, chilled
- 1-ounce Macadamia Nuts
- 1 tablespoon chia seeds
- 1 tablespoon MCT oil
- 1-2 packets Stevia, optional

Directions:
1. Add all the listed ingredients to a blender
2. Blend on high until smooth and creamy
3. Enjoy your smoothie!

Nutrition Info: Calories: 395; Fat: 39g; Carbohydrates: 11g; Protein: 5.2g

Great Nutty Lion

Servings: 2
Cooking Time: 5 Minutes
Ingredients:
- 1 tablespoon almond butter
- 1 tablespoon chia seeds
- 4 ice cubes
- ¾ cup plain low-fat Greek yogurt
- 1 cup baby spinach
- 1 cup unsweetened almond milk
- 2 fresh bananas

Directions:
1. Add all the ingredients except vegetables/fruits first
2. Blend until smooth
3. Add the vegetable/fruits
4. Blend until smooth
5. Add a few ice cubes and serve the smoothie
6. Enjoy!

Nutrition Info: Calories: 250; Fat: 10g; Carbohydrates: 51g; Protein: 8g

Muscular Macho Green

Servings: 2
Cooking Time: 5 Minutes
Ingredients:
- 2 teaspoons matcha powder
- 1 tablespoon chia seeds
- ¾ cup plain coconut yogurt
- 1 fresh banana
- 1 cup baby spinach
- 1 cup frozen mango
- 1 cup unsweetened coconut milk

Directions:
1. Add all the ingredients except vegetables/fruits first
2. Blend until smooth
3. Add the vegetable/fruits
4. Blend until smooth
5. Add a few ice cubes and serve the smoothie
6. Enjoy!

Nutrition Info: Calories: 200; Fat: 5g; Carbohydrates: 35g; Protein: 6g

Berry-celery Smoothie

Servings: 1 Large
Cooking Time: 2 Minutes
Ingredients:
- 1 cup blueberries (fresh or frozen)
- 2 medium peaches, pitted and chopped
- 1-2 stalk of celery, chopped
- 2 chard laves
- 1 teaspoon flaxseeds
- ½ teaspoon raw organic honey (optional)
- ½ cup filtered water
- 2-3 cubes of ice

Directions:
1. Load your high speed blender jar with the ingredients and run it on medium high sped for 30 seconds until a smooth, lump less mixture id obtained. Pour into serving glass and enjoy!

Nutrition Info: (Per Serving): Calories- 240, Fat- 1.54 g, Protein- 6.4 g, Carbohydrates- 48 g

Mango- Chia- Coconut Smoothie

Servings: 3
Cooking Time: 5 Minutes
Ingredients:
- 2 cups unsweetened organic coconut milk
- 1 cup mixed berries (fresh or frozen)
- 1 cup mango, chopped (fresh or frozen)

- 1 cup fresh kale, stems removed and chopped
- 1 large banana, chopped (fresh or frozen)
- 2 tablespoons Chia seeds, soaked
- 3 teaspoons of cashew butter
- ¼ cup of filtered water

Directions:
1. Add all the ingredients into the blender jar one by one, secure the lid firmly and whizz for 30 seconds or until done.

Nutrition Info: (Per Serving): Calories- 170, Fat- 6.8 g, Protein- 5 g, Carbohydrates- 25 g

Cheery Charlie Checker

Servings: 2
Cooking Time: 5 Minutes
Ingredients:
- 1 cup skim milk
- 1 cup frozen blueberries
- 1 fresh banana
- ¾ cup plain low-fat Greek yogurt
- ½ cup frozen cherries
- ½ cup frozen strawberries
- 1 tablespoon chia seeds

Directions:
1. Add all the ingredients except vegetables/fruits first
2. Blend until smooth
3. Add the vegetable/fruits
4. Blend until smooth
5. Add a few ice cubes and serve the smoothie
6. Enjoy!

Nutrition Info: Calories: 162; Fat: 1g; Carbohydrates: 33g; Protein: 8g

Beet-berry Brain Booster

Servings: 2
Cooking Time: 5 Minutes
Ingredients:
- 1/3 cup apple, cored and chopped
- ½ cup raw red beet, peeled and chopped
- 1 cup carrots, peeled and chopped
- ½ cup blueberries (fresh or frozen)
- 1 teaspoon freshly squeezed lemon juice
- 1/3 cup unsalted almonds
- ½ teaspoon freshly grated ginger
- 1 teaspoon raw organic honey
- A handful of ice cubes

Directions:

1. Load your blender with the ingredient listed above and process on medium high for 30 seconds or until done. Serve immediately.

Nutrition Info: (Per Serving): Calories- 322, Fat- 8 g, Protein- 11 g, Carbohydrates- 36 g

Nutty Bean "n"berry Smoothie

Servings: 2-3
Cooking Time: 5 Minutes
Ingredients:
- 1 cup blueberries (fresh or frozen)
- 1 cup whole strawberries (fresh or frozen)
- 1 large, raw brazil nut (roughly chopped)
- ½ cup cannellini beans (soaked overnight, drained and rinsed)
- 2 teaspoons sunflower seeds
- 2 teaspoon flax seed powder
- 1 ½ cups of filtered water

Directions:
1. Load your high speed blender jar with all the ingredients and puree until thick and smooth.

Nutrition Info: (Per Serving): Calories- 163, Fat- 6.4 g, Protein- 6.3 g, Carbohydrates- 23 g

BEAUTY SMOOTHIES

Cantaloupe Yogurt Smoothie

Servings: 1 Large
Cooking Time: 2 Minutes
Ingredients:
- 1 cup cantaloupe, chopped
- 1/3 cup plain yogurt
- ¼ teaspoon freshly grated ginger
- A pinch of nutmeg powder
- 1 tablespoon raw organic honey
- 1 teaspoon freshly squeezed lemon juice
- 3-4 mint leaves
- ½ cup filtered water
- 6-7 ice cubes

Directions:
1. Place everything into a blender and blitz until smooth. Pour into a glass and enjoy!

Nutrition Info: (Per Serving): Calories- 90, Fat- 0.9 g, Protein- 3.1 g, Carbohydrates- 20 g

Berry Beautiful Glowing Skin Smoothie

Servings: 2
Cooking Time: 5 Minutes
Ingredients:
- 1 cup blueberries (fresh or frozen)
- ½ cup raspberries (fresh or frozen)
- ½ cup strawberries (fresh or frozen)
- A handful of fresh kale, stems removed and chopped
- ¾ cup of plain Greek yogurt
- 2 teaspoon of raw organic honey
- 2 teaspoons freshly squeezed lemon juice
- 3 teaspoons flaxseed powder
- 4-5 ice cubes

Directions:
1. Pour all the ingredients into your blender and process until smooth.

Nutrition Info: (Per Serving): Calories- 161, Fat- 1.3 g, Protein- 8.9 g, Carbohydrates- 32 g

Chocolate Shake Smoothie

Servings: 2
Cooking Time: 5 Minutes
Ingredients:
- 1 ½ cups unsweetened almond milk
- 6 teaspoons raw organic cacao powder
- 4 tablespoons Chia seeds, soaked
- 1 teaspoon vanilla extract

- 5 teaspoons raw, organic honey
- A small pinch of cinnamon powder
- 3-4 ice cubes

Directions:

1. Combine all the ingredients in your high speed blender and puree until it is thick and creamy.

Nutrition Info: (Per Serving): Calories- 428, Fat- 15 g, Protein- 10 g, Carbohydrates- 70 g

Pink Potion

Servings: 3-4
Cooking Time: 5 Minutes

Ingredients:

- 2 cups raw beet, peeled and chopped
- 2 cups whole strawberries (fresh or frozen)
- 2 tablespoons almond butter
- 2 fresh kale leaves stems removed and chopped
- 1 banana, sliced (fresh or frozen)
- 1 teaspoon vanilla extract
- 1 tablespoon hemp seeds
- 1 cup filtered water

Directions:

1. Place all the ingredients into the blender and whiz up until the smoothie is nice and thick.

Nutrition Info: (Per Serving): Calories- 285, Fat- 11 g, Protein- 9.9 g, Carbohydrates- 40 g

All In 1 Smoothie

Servings: 2-3
Cooking Time: 5 Minutes

Ingredients:

- ½ cup freshly squeezed orange juice
- 1 cup carrots, peeled and chopped
- 1 cup fresh mixed greens of your choice
- 1 cup mixed berries (fresh or frozen)
- 1 small banana, copped (fresh or frozen)
- ½ cup plain low fat yogurt
- 2-3 drops of vanilla extract
- 1 teaspoon freshly squeezed lemon juice
- 3-4 ice cubes

Directions:

1. Pour all the ingredients into your blender and process until smooth.

Nutrition Info: (Per Serving): Calories- 160, Fat- 1.2 g, Protein- 5.3 g, Carbohydrates- 35 g

Orange- Green Tonic

Servings: 1 Large

Cooking Time: 2 Minutes
Ingredients:

- ¾ cup mango, chopped
- ½ cup freshly squeezed orange juice
- ¾ cup fresh kale, stems removed and chopped
- 1-2 celery stalks, chopped
- 2 tablespoons fresh parsley
- 5-6 fresh mint
- 4-5 ice cubes

Directions:

1. Just add all the ingredients into the blender, secure the lid and whizz it up until nice and smooth.

Nutrition Info: (Per Serving): Calories- 160, Fat- 0.7 g, Protein- 4.3 g, Carbohydrates- 38.5 g

Chocolaty Berry Blast

Servings: 2
Cooking Time: 2 Minutes
Ingredients:

- 2 cups unsweetened almond milk
- ½ cup Goji berries
- ½ cup whole almonds, soaked
- 6 teaspoons of raw cacao powder
- 1 tablespoon of raw organic honey
- 3-4 ice cubes

Directions:

1. To you blender, add all the above ingredient and pulse until smooth.

Nutrition Info: (Per Serving): Calories- 440, Fat- 23 g, Protein- 16 g, Carbohydrates- 43 g

Saffron Oats Smoothie

Servings: 2-3
Cooking Time: 5 Minutes
Ingredients:

- 2 ripe banana, sliced (fresh or frozen)
- 1 cup fresh coconut water
- 1 teaspoon raw organic honey
- 2 tablespoons oats
- ½ teaspoon vanilla extract
- A pinch of saffron
- ½ teaspoon of almond or cashew flakes (optional)

Directions:

1. Place everything in the blender jar, secure the lid and pulse until smooth.

Nutrition Info: (Per Serving): Calories- 136, Fat- 1.2 g, Protein- 1.3 g, Carbohydrates- 33 g

Bluberry Cucumber Cooler

Servings: 2
Cooking Time: 5 Minutes
Ingredients:
- 1 cup whole blueberries (fresh or frozen)
- 1 cup unsweetened almond milk
- ½ cup cucumber, chopped
- 2 large lettuce leaves
- 2 teaspoons hemp seeds
- 1 teaspoon raw organic honey (optional)
- 3-4 ice cubes

Directions:
1. Place all the ingredients into your blender and whirr it on high for 20 seconds or until the desired consistency has been reached. Pour into glasses and serve immediately.

Nutrition Info: (Per Serving): Calories- 202, Fat- 7.2 g, Protein- 6 g, Carbohydrates- 30 g

Aloe Berry Smoothie

Servings: 2
Cooking Time: 2 Minutes
Ingredients:
- ½ cup blueberries (fresh or frozen)
- 1/3 cup fresh and pure aloe gel or aloe Vera juice
- 2 tablespoons avocado flesh
- A handful of dandelion greens, chopped
- 1 kiwi, peeled and chopped
- 1 teaspoon coconut oil
- 1 teaspoon cacao powder
- A pinch of Celtic salt
- 1 ½ teaspoons of raw organic honey
- 1 cup filtered water

Directions:
1. Combine all the ingredients in a blender, secure the lid firmly and blitz until smooth.

Nutrition Info: (Per Serving): Calories- 305, Fat- 15 g, Protein- 2.1 g, Carbohydrates- 45 g

ENERGY BOOSTING SMOOTHIES

Grape And Green Tea Smoothie

Servings: 2-3
Cooking Time: 20 Minutes
Ingredients:
- 1 ½ cups freshly brewed green tea
- A handful of baby spinach, washed and chopped
- 1 cup kale, stems removed and chopped
- ½ cup green grapes(seedless)
- ½ avocado, peeled and chopped
- 1 ripe banana, chopped (fresh or frozen)
- 2 teaspoons Chia seeds, soaked for 15 minutes
- 2-3 ice cubes

Directions:
1.   Place all the items into the blender jar, secure the lid firmly and process until the smoothie has reached the desired consistency.

Nutrition Info: (Per Serving): Calories- 160, Fat- 6.7, Protein- 3.8 g, Carbohydrates- 20 g

Dandelion And Carrot Booster

Servings: 2
Cooking Time: 5 Minutes
Ingredients:
- ½ fuji apple
- 1 tablespoon fresh ginger
- ½ pound organic carrots, scrubbed
- ¾ cup dandelion greens
- 2 cups baby spinach

Directions:
1.   Add all the ingredients except vegetables/fruits first
2.   Blend until smooth
3.   Add the vegetable/fruits
4.   Blend until smooth
5.   Add a few ice cubes and serve the smoothie
6.   Enjoy!

Nutrition Info: Calories: 160; Fat: 5g; Carbohydrates: 30g; Protein: 5g

Verry- Berry Breakfast

Servings: 2
Cooking Time: 2 Minutes
Ingredients:
- ¾ cup unsweetened almond milk
- ½ large banana, chopped
- ¾ cup plain Greek yogurt

- 1 cup mixed berries (fresh or frozen)
- ½ teaspoon raw organic honey (optional)
- 3-5 ice cubes

Directions:
1. Place all the above ingredients into your high speed blender and process for 45 seconds on medium high speed till the smoothie is thick and creamy.

Nutrition Info: (Per Serving): Calories- 255, Fat- 1.2 g, Protein- 26 g, Carbohydrates- 42 g

Coconut- Flaxseed Smoothie

Servings: 1
Cooking Time: 2 Minutes
Ingredients:
- 1 cup fresh coconut water
- 1 small bananas, chopped
- 4 spinach leaves, washed and chopped
- ½ cup whole strawberries (fresh or frozen)
- 1 tablespoon flaxseed powder
- 3-4 ice cubes

Directions:
1. Load all the ingredients into the blender and whiz until smooth.

Nutrition Info: (Per Serving): Calories- 300, Fat- 4.2 g, Protein- 6.2 g, Carbohydrates- 67 g

Powerful Purple Smoothie

Servings: 2
Cooking Time: 5 Minutes
Ingredients:
- 1 tablespoon green superfood as you like
- 1 tablespoon spirulina
- 1 frozen banana, sliced
- 2 acai frozen berry packs
- 2 cups baby spinach
- 1¼ cups of coconut water

Directions:
1. Add all the ingredients except vegetables/fruits first
2. Blend until smooth
3. Add the vegetable/fruits
4. Blend until smooth
5. Add a few ice cubes and serve the smoothie
6. Enjoy!

Nutrition Info: Calories: 70; Fat: 2g; Carbohydrates: 14g; Protein: 3g

Generous Mango Surprise

Servings: 2
Cooking Time: 5 Minutes
Ingredients:
- 1 tablespoon spirulina
- 3 cups frozen mango, sliced
- 1½ cups kale
- 2½ cups unsweetened almond milk

Directions:
1. Add all the ingredients except vegetables/fruits first
2. Blend until smooth
3. Add the vegetable/fruits
4. Blend until smooth
5. Add a few ice cubes and serve the smoothie
6. Enjoy!

Nutrition Info: Calories: 72; Fat: 0g; Carbohydrates: 17g; Protein: 1g

Cinnamon Mango Smoothie

Servings: 2
Cooking Time: 10 Minutes
Ingredients:
- 2 mangoes, peeled, pit removed and chopped
- ½ teaspoon cinnamon, grounded
- 2 teaspoons lime juice
- 2 cups plain yogurt, low-fat
- 1 tablespoon honey

Directions:
1. Add all the listed ingredients to a blender
2. Blend until you have a smooth and creamy texture
3. Serve chilled and enjoy!

Nutrition Info: Calories: 210; Fat: 2.2g; Carbohydrates: 40.2g; Protein: 8.5g

Powerful Green Frenzy

Servings: 2
Cooking Time: 5 Minutes
Ingredients:
- 1 cup ice
- 2 tablespoons almond butter
- 1 teaspoon spirulina
- 3 teaspoons fresh ginger
- 1½ frozen bananas, sliced
- 2 cups baby spinach, chopped
- 1 cup kale

- 1½ cups unsweetened almond milk

Directions:
1. Add all the ingredients except vegetables/fruits first
2. Blend until smooth
3. Add the vegetable/fruits
4. Blend until smooth
5. Add a few ice cubes and serve the smoothie
6. Enjoy!

Nutrition Info: Calories: 350; Fat: 4g; Carbohydrates: 54g; Protein: 30g

Berry- Mint Cooler

Servings: 2
Cooking Time: 2 Minutes
Ingredients:
- 2 cups unsweetened almond milk
- A large handful of frozen blueberries
- 1 ½ teaspoons of raw, organic honey
- 1 ½ teaspoon flax seed powder
- 3-4 fresh mint leaves
- 4-5 ice cubes

Directions:
1. To your high speed blender, add all the ingredients and process for 30 seconds or until done.

Nutrition Info: (Per Serving): Calories- 201, Fat-7.2 g, Protein-11 g, Carbohydrates- 21 g

Green Skinny Energizer

Servings: 2
Cooking Time: 5 Minutes
Ingredients:
- ½ ripe mango, pitted and sliced
- 1 cup kale, chopped
- 3 cups baby spinach
- 1 cup coconut water

Directions:
1. Add all the ingredients except vegetables/fruits first
2. Blend until smooth
3. Add the vegetable/fruits
4. Blend until smooth
5. Add a few ice cubes and serve the smoothie
6. Enjoy!

Nutrition Info: Calories: 300; Fat: 13g; Carbohydrates: 37g; Protein: 10g

Servings: 2
Cooking Time: 5 Minutes
Ingredients:
- 1 persimmon, topped and chopped
- 1 tablespoon cinnamon
- 1 squash
- 1 tablespoon flaxseed
- 4 ounces pineapple
- 1 tablespoon pea protein
- 1 cup of water

Directions:
1. Add all the listed ingredients to a blender
2. Blend until you have a smooth and creamy texture
3. Serve chilled and enjoy!

Nutrition Info: Calories: 159; Fat: 2g; Carbohydrates: 33g; Protein: 7g

DIABETES SMOOTHIES

Berry Truffle Smoothie

Servings: 2
Cooking Time: 10 Minutes
Ingredients:
- 1 medium Haas avocado
- 1 and ¼ teaspoons pure vanilla extract
- ½ cup whipping cream
- 3 tablespoons cocoa powder, unsweetened
- 4 tablespoons pecans
- 1 and ¼ cups mixed berries, frozen
- 2 pinches salt
- ¾ cups of ice cubes
- Erythritol, to taste
- 1 cup of water

Directions:
1. Add all the listed ingredients to a blender
2. Blend until you have a smooth and creamy texture
3. Serve chilled and enjoy!

Nutrition Info: Calories: 375; Fat: 32.5g; Carbohydrates: 11.3g; Protein: 5.8g

Pineapple Broccoli Smoothie

Servings: 2
Cooking Time: 10 Minutes
Ingredients:
- 1 cup strawberries
- 2 cups almond milk
- 2 cups broccoli florets
- ½ cup pineapple
- 2 teaspoons honey

Directions:
1. Add listed ingredients to a blender
2. Blend until you have a smooth and creamy texture
3. Serve chilled and enjoy!

Nutrition Info: Calories: 324; Fat: 25.4g; Carbohydrates: 18g; Protein: 4.3g

Avocado And Edamame Drink

Servings: 2
Cooking Time: 5 Minutes
Ingredients:
- ¾ cup almond milk
- ½ cup edamame shelled
- ¼ cup avocado, diced
- ½ cup of frozen mango, diced

- 1 tablespoon coconut flour
- 1 cup ice

Directions:
1. Add all the ingredients except vegetables/fruits first
2. Blend until smooth
3. Add the vegetable/fruits
4. Blend until smooth
5. Add a few ice cubes and serve the smoothie
6. Enjoy!

Nutrition Info: Calories: 245; Fat: 15g; Carbohydrates: 28g; Protein: 4g

Peanut Butter And Raspberry Delight

Servings: 2
Cooking Time: 5 Minutes
Ingredients:
- 1 tablespoon psyllium husk
- 1 tablespoon unsweetened peanut butter
- 2 tablespoons powdered peanut butter
- ¾ cup frozen cherries
- ½ cup silken tofu
- ¾ cup non-fat milk such as almond milk

Directions:
1. Add all the ingredients except vegetables/fruits first
2. Blend until smooth
3. Add the vegetable/fruits
4. Blend until smooth
5. Add a few ice cubes and serve the smoothie
6. Enjoy!

Nutrition Info: Calories: 170; Fat: 8g; Carbohydrates: 24g; Protein: 6g

Keto Mocha Smoothie

Servings: 4
Cooking Time: 10 Minutes
Ingredients:
- 6 tablespoons cocoa powder, unsweetened
- 1 cup of coconut milk
- 3 cups almond milk, unsweetened
- 2 avocados, cut in half
- 2 teaspoons vanilla extract
- 6 tablespoons erythritol, granulated
- 4 teaspoons instant coffee crystals

Directions:
1. Add all the listed ingredients to a blender
2. Blend until you have a smooth and creamy texture
3. Serve chilled and enjoy!

Nutrition Info: Calories: 273; Fat: 24.3g; Carbohydrates: 8.2g; Protein: 4.5g

Strawberry – Banana Smoothie

Servings: 2
Cooking Time: 5 Minutes
Ingredients:
- 2 small heads of bok choy
- 2 cups whole strawberries (fresh or frozen)
- 1 large banana, chopped (fresh or frozen)
- 2 tablespoon avocado flesh
- 1 teaspoon flax seed powder
- ½ cup filtered water

Directions:
1. Combine all the ingredients in the blender and pulse until smooth

Nutrition Info: (Per Serving): Calories- 290, Fat- 10 g, Protein- 6.2 g, Carbohydrates- 55 g

Tropical Kiwi Pineapple

Servings: 2
Cooking Time: 5 Minutes
Ingredients:
- 1 cup ice
- 1 tablespoon ground flaxseed
- 1 tablespoon psyllium husk
- 6 almonds
- 2 tablespoons unsweetened coconut
- 1 medium kiwi, skin intact

Directions:
1. Add all the ingredients except vegetables/fruits first
2. Blend until smooth
3. Add the vegetable/fruits
4. Blend until smooth
5. Add a few ice cubes and serve the smoothie
6. Enjoy!

Nutrition Info: Calories: 300; Fat: 15g; Carbohydrates: 40g; Protein: 1g

Apple- Yogurt Green Smoothie

Servings: 2
Cooking Time: 5 Minutes
Ingredients:
- 1 large apple, cored and chopped
- 2 cups of plain Greek yogurt
- 1 cup fresh baby spinach, washed and chopped
- 2 teaspoons of freshly squeezed lemon juice

- 1 teaspoon flaxseed powder

Directions:

1. Pour the liquids, apples, spinach and flax seed powder into the blender Jar and puree until thick and creamy.

Nutrition Info: (Per Serving): Calories- 165, Fat- 5, Protein- 10 g, Carbohydrates- 33 g

Lime "n" Lemony Cucumber Cooler

Servings: 3

Cooking Time: 5 Minutes

Ingredients:

- 2 cups plain fat free yogurt
- 2 cups green cucumber, chopped
- 1 green pear, cored and chopped
- Freshly squeezed juice of 1 lime
- 1 tablespoon freshly squeezed lemon juice
- 2-3 ice cubes

Directions:

1. Place all the ingredients into the high speed blender and blitz until thick and creamy. Serve immediately!

Nutrition Info: (Per Serving): Calories- 175, Fat- 4.2 g, Protein- 11 g, Carbohydrates- 63 g

Choco Spinach Delight

Servings: 1

Cooking Time: 10 Minutes

Ingredients:

- 4 ice cubes
- 1 scoop green superfood
- 1 scoop protein powder
- 1 tablespoon chia seeds
- ½ cup berry yogurt
- 1 handful of organic spinach
- 1 teaspoon organic flaxseed
- ½ avocado
- 1/3 cup organic strawberries, frozen
- ½ cup organic blueberries, frozen
- ¾ cup unsweetened almond milk

Directions:

1. Add all the listed ingredients to a blender
2. Blend until you have a smooth and creamy texture
3. Serve chilled and enjoy!

Nutrition Info: Calories: 180; Fat: 16g; Carbohydrates: 7g; Protein: 1g

Servings: 2
Cooking Time: 5 Minutes
Ingredients:
- 1 cup ice
- 2 tablespoons fresh mint leaves, chopped
- 1 tablespoon coconut flour
- 2 tablespoons hemp seeds
- ½ cup frozen spinach
- ½ cup frozen mango
- 1/3 cup white beans, rinsed
- 1 cup cashew milk

Directions:
1. Add all the ingredients except vegetables/fruits first
2. Blend until smooth
3. Add the vegetable/fruits
4. Blend until smooth
5. Add a few ice cubes and serve the smoothie
6. Enjoy!

Nutrition Info: Calories: 290; Fat: 10g; Carbohydrates: 37g; Protein: 12g

Printed by BoD™in Norderstedt, Germany